The Kawa Model

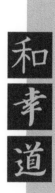

To Occupational Therapy Practitioners,

for in your hands lies the essence of culturally relevant occupational therapy

To the memory of Professor Tsuyoshi Sato

For Elsevier:

Commissioning Editor: Susan Young

Development Editor: Catherine Jackson

Project Manager: Gail Wright

Designer: Stewart Larking

Illustration Buyer: Merlyn Harvey

Illustrator: Richard Morris

The Kawa Model

Culturally Relevant Occupational Therapy

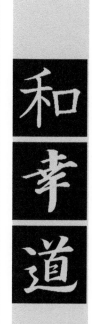

Michael K. Iwama
PhD MSc BScOT BSc

Associate Professor,
Department of Occupational Science and Occupational
Therapy, Faculty of Medicine,
University of Toronto, Toronto, ON, Canada

Forewords by

M. Carolyn Baum
PhD OTR/L FAOTA

Professor of Occupational Therapy
and Professor of Neurology, and Elias Michael Director,
Program in Occupational Therapy, Washington University
School of Medicine, St Louis, MO, USA

and

Charles Christiansen
EDD OTR OT(C) FAOTA

Dean and Professor, School of Allied Health Sciences,
George T. Bryan Distinguished Professor,
University of Texas Medical Branch, Galveston, Texas, USA

EDINBURGH LONDON NEW YORK OXFORD PHILADELPHIA ST LOUIS SYDNEY TORONTO 2006

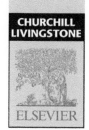

CHURCHILL LIVINGSTONE
ELSEVIER

© 2006, Elsevier Limited. All rights reserved.

No part of this publication may be reproduced, stored in a retrieval system, or transmitted in any form or by any means, electronic, mechanical, photocopying, recording or otherwise, without the prior permission of the Publishers. Permissions may be sought directly from Elsevier's Health Sciences Rights Department, 1600 John F. Kennedy Boulevard, Suite 1800, Philadelphia, PA 19103-2899, USA: phone: (+1) 215 239 3804; fax: (+1) 215 239 3805; or, e-mail: *healthpermissions@elsevier.com*. You may also complete your request on-line via the Elsevier homepage (http://www.elsevier.com), by selecting 'Support and contact' and then 'Copyright and Permission'.

First published 2006

ISBN-13: 978-0-443-10234-9
ISBN-10: 0 443 10234 1

British Library Cataloguing in Publication Data
A catalogue record for this book is available from the British Library

Library of Congress Cataloging in Publication Data
A catalog record for this book is available from the Library of Congress

Note
Knowledge and best practice in this field are constantly changing. As new research and experience broaden our knowledge, changes in practice, treatment and drug therapy may become necessary or appropriate. Readers are advised to check the most current information provided (i) on procedures featured or (ii) by the manufacturer of each product to be administered, to verify the recommended dose or formula, the method and duration of administration, and contraindications. It is the responsibility of the practitioner, relying on their own experience and knowledge of the patient, to make diagnoses, to determine dosages and the best treatment for each individual patient, and to take all appropriate safety precautions. To the fullest extent of the law, neither the Publisher nor the Author assumes any liability for any injury and/or damage to persons or property arising out or related to any use of the material contained in this book.

The Publisher

ELSEVIER your source for books, journals and multimedia in the health sciences
www.elsevierhealth.com

Working together to grow libraries in developing countries

www.elsevier.com | www.bookaid.org | www.sabre.org

ELSEVIER   BOOK AID International   Sabre Foundation

Printed and bound by CPI Group (UK) Ltd, Croydon, CR0 4YY

Transferred to digital print 2013

The publisher's policy is to use paper manufactured from sustainable forests

Contents 川

Foreword 川

M. Carolyn Baum

Each of us has had a chance meeting that has had a major impact on our life. I had such an experience in September 2003 in the San Francisco airport. A young man came up to me and said 'Dr Baum, may I have the privilege of accompanying you to Singapore?' That young man was Michael Iwama and it was serendipity that we were scheduled on the same plane en route to Singapore for the 3rd Asia Pacific Occupational Therapy Congress.

For the next 16 hours I was captivated by a young man with commitment to the profession and its history. He had a knowledge of theory, social context and culture and a passion to help us all to understand and then implement programs and services that cross cultural boundaries. His message was that because we focus on the daily lives of people we must understand and respect not only the culture of nations but also the cultural diversity within the boundaries of our own communities and organizations in which people live and work. My life was changed, as my view of occupational therapy in the world was expanded and I saw a young scholar who would make a contribution not only to our profession but to the world.

In this book Dr Iwama challenges us to expand our minds and actions beyond our own social boundaries to those that our clients find meaningful. He asks us to look at the lived and socially constructed experiences of the people we serve rather than hold on to those with which we are comfortable.

This is a very important book for both teachers and students of occupational therapy. Dr Iwama helps us define the culture of occupational therapy by exploring its theory, constructs and principles. He challenges us to look beyond our own knowledge and experience and to place that knowledge in the context in which it is applied – in the lives of people as they address problems that limit their daily activities. He supports the reader as they accept this challenge. As he gives life to the concepts, he gives us ideas to discuss and, most importantly, he

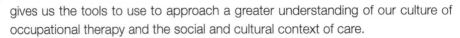
gives us the tools to use to approach a greater understanding of our culture of occupational therapy and the social and cultural context of care.

Most of the occupational therapy models in use today, including The Person-Environment-Occupational-Performance Model developed by my colleague Charles Christiansen and me, are informed by common experience situated in the Western world. We cannot assume that these models are universally appropriate as we see occupational therapy continue its growth around the world (currently there are 60 member countries in the World Federation of Occupational Therapists, many in developing countries). There is a specific need to have contemporary models to meet diverse social contexts.

The Kawa model is an exemplar of how occupational therapy can fit the people it will serve. Although I was introduced to the model from the Japanese perspective I find myself thinking a lot about it because of the way the Kawa model encourages us to see disability and chronic disease as a collective experience. It asks us to view the self as a number of elements that cannot be separated. These elements include life circumstances, strengths and limitations and life flow, which includes goals, relationships and health.

I grew up in a faming community in Kansas. Recently I was explaining what occupational therapists do to a friend from my home town. Because he is a farmer and very passionate about his land I used the Kawa model to explain how rocks and roots of trees can block the flow of a stream. When we discussed what those blocks to the stream might be I explained to him what the OT could do to help the person 'restore the flow of the stream'. He was very interested in what I do and he understood it because I explained it in a context that was understandable to him.

I want to share one more experience that shows the strength of the Kawa model. Recently I got a call from the Dean of Medicine's office asking if I could speak to a visitor from Japan. He was planning a visit by Japanese medical students to learn about advances in Western medicine. He arrived expecting to talk about physical therapy and when I told him I was director of occupational therapy he looked as if he wanted to leave, saying that he wanted his students to learn about advances in physical rehabilitation. I pointed out that some of the most important work in the development of contemporary rehabilitation is being developed by occupational therapists in Japan and told him a little about the Kawa model.

He mentioned that Kawa means river in Japanese and I explained that the river serves as a metaphor to let the patient (he was a doctor so I used the term patient) share the experience that is causing the difficulties that require rehabilitation. We then went on to speak about why occupational therapy is essential to helping people overcome problems that threaten their health and well-being.

I told him about our innovative community programs and he then decided that he definitely wanted his students to learn about occupational therapy during their visit to the medical school. He also asked if he could take away some information about the Kawa model, which I was very pleased to provide.

We need tools to work with those who need our services and to communicate our uniqueness to others. I believe the Kawa model can help us focus our work on individuals in the context of their lives.

Dr Iwama's book will give us knowledge and it challenges us to think about the culture of our profession as well as the culture of those with whom we work. It will also help us gain insight into the cultures of organizations and groups.

This book should form the basis of theory courses for students around the world – the discussions that will ensue will go a long way to helping us understand that in fact the world is flat and that occupational therapists all over the world can learn from each other because we share a culture of occupational therapy. The book will also help us all honor the cultures of the people we serve as we seek to improve their everyday lives.

Foreword
Charles Christiansen

There is a Japanese concept, expressed in the word *nyuanshin*, which describes a readiness to learn. This 'beginner's mind', openly receptive to new ideas, is an excellent state from which to begin exploring this book, particularly if one is a reader grounded in Western ideas about occupational therapy.

In the parlance of science, sets of ideas about phenomena are variously called paradigms, models, frameworks or theories. These sets of ideas represent particular ways of viewing the world and its events. Michael Iwama points out that these world views, or ways of thinking, are very much influenced by the shared meanings ascribed to phenomena that have been constructed within a particular culture. The forming of these views can come from tradition, expert consensus, empirical research or some combination of these processes. Regardless of how they evolve, shared meanings and explanations that make the world of practice comprehensible are so much a part of our everyday interpretations of experience that we seldom think about them and even less frequently question them. As the author points out in *The Kawa Model*, this can be problematic for many reasons.

The late Thomas Kuhn, historian and observer of science, described the progress of science as something that was far less linear and more social and political than non-scientists might take comfort in believing[1]. Practitioners or technologists who use frameworks as guides for applying knowledge in their daily work seldom readily embrace new frameworks, however well crafted. This is because the status quo is comfortable and familiar, and also because those who established the prevailing ways of looking at the world want them to remain dominant, regardless of the potential benefits conferred by adopting a new viewpoint. Self-interest, cultivated through a career-long process of gaining acceptance of a particular point of view, sometimes makes it difficult for the advocates of a new framework to persuade others of its merits. In short, there are forces at play besides the intrinsic benefits of a new model that may work against its adoption. As a consequence, noted Kuhn, new ideas in the scientific realm have to be pretty good to get people's attention, and even better to become adopted widely enough to replace existing orthodoxies. For these reasons, the emergence of new world views creates unrest and upheaval. Perhaps this is why Kuhn described such events as *revolutions*.

It may be begging the question to assert that the ideas presented in this book constitute the beginning of a revolution. Yet there are many reasons why the Kawa model can claim to be an important development in the way occupational therapy is conceptualized. It is true that the model works better for people in cultures where collectivist rather than individual views of the world predominate; where interdependence rather than independence are the cornerstones of being; and where holistic, rather than reductionistic explanations of phenomena are seen as natural and more fitting.

Yet I believe the Kawa model will have intuitive appeal to many people in the West, because it is a wonderful and dynamic metaphor for life and the complexities of life's challenges. Like the flow of life itself, the model is fluid and as such, lends itself well to the subjective nature of human experience. The popular US writer, lecturer and student of Eastern religions, Alan Watts, noted that the world, after all, is not constructed of straight lines. He observed that nature does very well in creating harmony and beauty with irregular, curved or squiggly lines – precisely the kind found in drawings of water, or rivers[2].

And so it is that the Kawa model, by drawing from nature, does such an effective job of providing a metaphor for the vicissitudes of life. In so doing it provides a readily understandable way for both practitioners and clients (be they individuals or collectives) to understand what occupational therapy is trying to achieve as a service aimed at engendering participation, health and well-being. More importantly, this different way of understanding should more readily enable clients and practitioners alike to become engaged in the process of finding creative, appropriate and contextually relevant ways of dealing with those life challenges that create the need for intervention. This is genuine client-centred therapy at its best, where therapists empower clients to call upon their *ryuboku* (or personal characteristics and assets) within the context of their *torimaki* (physical and social environment) with an eye toward using *sukima* (occupations) to contend with the *iwa* (circumstances) that impede their life course.

It is not surprising, given the Japanese roots of the Kawa model, that there are abundant similarities between its concepts and precepts of Zen Buddhism and Taoism. René Descartes, the 17th-century French mathematician, scientist and philosopher, is credited with many important ideas that have contributed to the advancement of civilization[3]. However, his insistence upon interpreting and understanding only a world that could be observed and measured helped contribute to the reductionistic approaches that have dominated so much of science in the past and present. This obsession with the quantifiable and reductionistic as the predominate ways of knowing has also been blamed (using Phillip Shannon's words) for the historical derailment of occupational therapy[4]. When occupational therapists are content with addressing impairments without consideration of their impact on the lives of their clients, they are using a model of intervention that is unrelated to the founding ideas of the field. Sadly, remnants of the wreckage of occupational therapy's derailment continue to litter the professional landscape.

With this book, and its ability to more broadly share the beauty of the Kawa model with the English-speaking countries of the West, Michael Iwama has delivered a gift to the profession. At the very least, it will sensitize readers to the reality of how cultural differences shape ways of knowing. It has the potential, however, to do much more. It provides a way of understanding occupational therapy in the context of lives that makes it nearly impossible for one exposed to its fluidity to ever view therapy in quite the same way again.

There has been a tension in occupational therapy between its qualitative nature and its existence in a scientific world that values quantitative and positivistic demonstrations of 'truth'. This tension is aggravated in the current outcome-oriented, cost-conscious, evidence-driven milieu of health care in the USA[5]. As so many have stated, however, occupational therapy is almost uniquely a profession where the worlds of applied science and lived experience have been able to come together. As Tristram Englehardt[6] so richly described it, occupational therapists are both technologists *and* custodians of meaning. Too often, these days, too much attention is given to the human as body rather than the human as *being*. The Kawa model, used alongside Western models of occupational therapy (with their tendency toward straight-line orientations), will enable a more balanced understanding of how occupational therapy should be practised. In so doing, it will add value to the way we think about clients and, thus, enrich the relevance and outcomes of occupational therapy services provided for them.

REFERENCES

[1] Kuhn T. The structure of scientific revolutions. Chicago: University of Chicago Press; 1962

[2] Watts AW. Tao: The Watercourse Way. New York: Pantheon; 1975

[3] Doney W. Descartes: A Collection of Critical Essays. New York: Doubleday; 1967

[4] Shannon PD. The derailment of occupational therapy. American Journal of Occupational Therapy 1977; 31:229–234

[5] Mattingly C, Fleming M. Clinical reasoning. Philadelphia: FA Davis; 1993

[6] Englehardt HT. Occupational therapists as technologists and custodians of meaning. In: Kielhofner GW (ed.) Health through Occupation: Theory and Practice in Occupational Therapy. Philadelphia: FA Davis; 1983

川

Foreword

Preface 川

The promise of occupational therapy has always been a simple yet potentially powerful one – to enable people from all walks of life to perform meaningful activities. Fidler, Reilly, Yerxa, Wilcock, Baum, Townsend and a progression of the profession's visionaries have guided us along the most compelling aspect of occupational therapy's ideology, despite the enormous pressures that continue to confine our professional mandate within the modern biomedical paradigm. Their prophetic declarations about the essentiality of occupation, and the belief that one's engagement in meaningful and purposeful doing is profoundly tied to matters of human health and well-being, remain credible and resonate with a vast number of people who share the same contexts of experience and meaning; however, the assumptions about occupation and the relevance of occupational therapy, which take on universal qualities, remain largely unquestioned and rarely challenged.

While the concept of occupation and ideology of occupational therapy appear to resonate with many people situated in the normal social boundaries of middle North America, they may not, in their current constructions, resonate as strongly and as meaningfully with people abiding in other, differing, social contexts. My own experience, of acculturating into different ethnically and geographically located experiences at various points in my life, has stimulated thoughts around the questions: how are ideas founded in one ('Western') perspective of the world adequate to explain and guide occupational therapy interventions for those who abide in another very different (cultural) reality? What does it mean for occupational therapists to mandate independence to collectively oriented, interdependent-conscious clients?

If we have not already asked it in our ever-increasing diverse practices, these are questions we will all need to ask eventually as occupational therapy finds its way across cultural boundaries within and outside of our national contexts of daily life. Although we frequently construe culture to traverse geographic locations and treat it as a static attribute located within the individual, we may need to expand culture to include spheres of experience (transcending the individual into the social realm) and consider how these individual markers of distinction are created and ascribed through a social dynamic. Taking it in this way, we need not cast our gazes to other nations and geographical locations, but examine the cultural diversity within the boundaries of our own communities where we live and practise. A broader regard for culture would take into account and foster an appreciation of other common spheres of experience around, for example, socio-economic groupings, political activity, gender, sexual orientation, religion and faith, or institutional life. All of these somewhat arbitrary and socially constructed categories (often reified by expansive products of the scientific academe) speak to different spheres of shared experience and represent their own developed values, social norms, rituals, etc.

Our clients in occupational therapy represent a constellation of uniquely lived and socially constructed spheres of experiences, yet we hold onto universal narratives of occupation and occupational therapy and even those perspectives borrowed from the culture of medicine, and proceed to translate these imperatives onto our unwitting and often vulnerable clients. This is perpetuated when we rarely question or critically examine the veracity and cultural safety of our theory, knowledge and methods in this still-fledgling profession, and when we push forward with our protocols without much regard to whether what we do has any real relevance with the client's contexts of daily realities. How client-centred are we being when we end up taking responses to our own constructed questions based on a particular construal of occupation and transform the responses we hear from our clients into the present culturally narrow lanes of occupational therapy ideology, texts and instruments?

Perhaps that is more of a commentary of where we have come from and where we are at this present time than it is about where this promising profession is progressing. Our theoretical materials and epistemology have yet to move through the post-modern and post-structural bumps and grinds that will take us from the rational and universal towards the culturally relative and culturally safe. Occupational therapists will need to figure out what to do with a heavily biomedical-influenced mandate based on physical evidence and pathology, or a mandate on Western, existentially situated views embodied in terms like self-efficacy, personal causation, occupational performance, self-care, productivity and leisure, for a global diverse clientele.

Occupational therapy has at times been classified as a *white middle class women's* profession. That classification is debatable and troublesome (and excluding for men of colour like me), but even more so when considered from the vantage of diverse societies that could benefit from occupational therapy. This profession's hidden power has been in its mandate to be relevant to the functions of daily life that we (society) often take for granted until we are either denied such functions or lose the ability to perform them. But our practice, knowledge and theory have sorely been lost on the needs of a diverse clientele who represent diverse spheres of experience outside the boundaries of occupational therapy's grand narratives. It has also placed occupational therapists like my (male) self, belonging to non-Western ethnic traditions, out towards the periphery. Perhaps we can point towards the funding structures, political conditions and institutional constraints of the world of medicine, to which we have been almost inextricably tied, that constrain and shape our practice; but perhaps it could also be that occupational therapists have been theoretically juvenile in not developing our materials and knowledge in a more culturally inclusive and socially equitable direction.

Those of us who have experienced a life and spheres of experience different to those that are reflected in contemporary occupational therapy have at times felt marginalised or uncomfortable about the processes that we engage in this profession. It has been challenging to call occupational therapy our own when much of it fails to resonate on a more profound, cultural level. Those of us who have not departed for other vocations will have questioned where the voices and representations of everyday life of our own cultures have been in occupational therapy. We aren't quite there yet, in contributing to our literature or to our leadership.

Yet we hold on to the hope that eventually our profession will move towards a more inclusive perspective. Occupational therapy has always been about enabling people to perform meaningful activities in daily life. There is tremendous power in this simple mandate. This promise is what holds me here and impels me to exert a view to move my chosen profession closer to this wonderful ideal. At this present time, the narratives, means and explanations of what this is are Western-centric and exclude a large majority of occupational therapy's clients and practitioners. Just ask anyone on the street what occupational therapy is and you'll see what I mean. Ask an occupational therapist in a non-English-language setting what the occupation in occupational therapy means and you are sure to get a variety of definitions – some wrong perhaps from your particular vantage.

This book is as much about honouring and respecting different cultural constructions of occupational therapy as it is about a model that serves as an example of an alternative view of the meanings of doing. It is a tool to be adapted and manipulated to suit the language and experience of occupation in varying cultural situations – not to translate our clients' experiences into a particular ethnocentric narrative. By respecting and giving credence to our clients' diverse views of reality and the meanings of doing in everyday life, we bring ourselves to a place where we consider reconceptualising occupation. The consequence of adopting this line of thinking and values shift is the creation of more concepts and alternate ideals – ideals that resonate meaningfully with the daily life experiences of *all* those we endeavour to serve.

A concern for this profession lies in the maintenance of ideals and concepts that are out of sync with our clients' real worlds of meaning. A profession that places the blinkers on alternative views and constructions of meaning in daily life stands to trivialise itself into extinction, and thus fall far short of occupational therapy's magnificent promise.

Michael K. Iwama
Okayama, Toronto, Brisbane 2006

CHAPTER 1

Situating Occupational Therapy's Knowledge

Why Alternative Conceptualisations and Models of Occupational Therapy Are Required

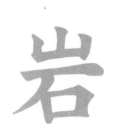

岩

Does contemporary occupational therapy theory harmonise with and adequately explain the contexts and shared experiences in the daily lives of occupational therapists and their clients? In this opening chapter, this fundamental issue of meaning in our profession is raised. *Meaning* of the core concepts of occupational therapy, the principles rationally connecting them, and the theoretical materials that follow are critically examined. This fundamental issue is often overlooked, yet has enormous bearing on whether occupational therapy is truly relevant, useful, fair and inclusive. In scientific language, we might say that we are examining matters of *construct validity* – whether the constructs and concepts being considered truly represent what they purport to. In the context of occupational therapy practice we might conduct such an examination by asking critical questions such as: whose ideas of occupation are these?; where did these ideas come from?; what influenced these ideas?; and do these ideas resonate with and agree in meaning with our clients' worlds of experiences?

Academicians are challenged to consider the validity of their theory, their constructs and principles and the veracity with which we regard the knowledge that informs and translates our theory into occupational therapy practice. Practitioners are challenged to look beyond the form of occupational therapy, as they have learned and practised it, towards a more comprehensive examination of the contexts in which their occupational therapy is applied. Occupational therapists are encouraged to examine critically whether their current occupational therapy is meaningful relative to the meanings of their clients' day-to-day realities.

We proceed directly, then, to the issue of why we need other conceptual models, like the Kawa[1] model, and why the profession of occupational therapy, for the sake of our clients, must critically consider the cultural dimensions[2] of its theory, models, knowledge base and patterns of practice. To deny this need is to overlook culture's fundamental importance to occupational therapy and to maintain certain exclusionary qualities of our profession which, in its current state, appears to favour the maintenance of normal Western world views and its modal spheres of experience. It is this current state that draws an inference that competing views of truth and occupation, which are situated outside its constructed boundaries of normal, require correction and cultivation. If occupational therapy is to become the relevant, powerful and useful entity that it can be, then the consideration of culturally relevant theoretical material and practice approaches is fundamental. A culturally inclusive occupational therapy is imperative.

What does *culture* have to do with the knowledge and theory of occupational therapy? And why do we need yet another conceptual model to describe, explain and guide our practice? The answers to these fundamental questions depend on how we define and regard culture, and whether we understand *culture* as a static feature of individuals – of occupational therapy clients and of their therapists – or as something much larger and pervasive, transcending the individual, to the broader processes that define the profession and practice of occupational therapy. How we orient ourselves to these fundamental questions may well determine whether our occupational therapy is truly as meaningful, relevant and helpful to our clients as we believe it to be.

Few of us are used to regarding occupational therapy as a cultural entity – a significant oversight in our profession's demonstrated views of culture – and this has limited our appreciation for its fundamental place in the form, function and meaning of occupation and occupational therapy. If we are serious about advancing this profession in a more culturally inclusive direction, and thereby increasing its meaningfulness and value to our clients and to society, then we must take a more critical perspective in evaluating the cultural norms that bind, shape and determine the relevance and meaning of occupational therapy to the social contexts in which we practise. And, rather than projecting our culturally bound narratives onto clients who may not abide in our own situated views of normal, we may need to develop and implement better ways for our clients' narratives to form the bases to our theory and knowledge, and direct the processes of occupational therapy.

Ideas and truth are given power by the social contexts from which they arise and wherein they reside. The particular world views informed by the collective experiences we share within groups are evident in our theories and ideas of occupation and the meanings that are ascribed to *doing*. These ideas do not flow from a vacuum nor from heaven but rather, they are thought up and expressed by human beings who are reflecting on what they believe to be true, worth knowing and worth doing. And these truths are, arguably, fundamentally grounded in common social spheres of experience. Whether we realise it or not, our conceptual models in occupational therapy are constructed in particular (Western) cultural contexts and reflect the world views, value patterns and perspectives of truth of their authors. We have not really made it a priority to recognise and understand the situated-ness of our knowledge, theory and practice. Subsequently, little heed is paid to the consequences that occur when the situated grand narratives of occupational therapy and the situated narratives of the client are out of sync.

When conceptual models are used in the same or similar cultural contexts in which they have been formed (or constructed), there exists greater probability for the model's inner concepts and the principles that bind them, and the overall structure in which they are organised, to resonate with the clients' real world of day-to-day experiences and meanings. Most of our current models of occupation and occupational therapy have been raised and informed by people who share common experiences and common views of truth, situated in the Western world – particularly urban North America. And we are probably mistaken if we assume that these views of reality are universally appropriate to explain the realities of occupational therapy's diverse clientele.

Independence fostered by a greater sense of individual determinism, rational thinking that gives order and a certain confidence in matters of time use and self-efficacy, and the celebration of the self as rational 'doer', are some of the common social features and value patterns that are evident in the profession's current epistemology and theory. What happens to these ideas, theoretical frameworks and emergent intervention designs when they cross cultural boundaries of meaning? Do the ideas, value patterns and views of reality embedded in the models transfer and integrate well with people representing all walks of life in your own communities? How do the discourses around occupation – of people as reflective, agent, *occupational beings*, as rational occupiers of environments, etc. – relate to people who abide outside of these culturally situated perspectives? Are the daily life patterns and meanings ascribed to doing of the elderly, children, of people living in conditions of poverty and disadvantage, diverse ethnic groups, including the aboriginal peoples of your nations, truly being appreciated and enabled by our contemporary theoretical frameworks?

A myriad of consequences surfaces when theory is out of sync and out of touch with practice and the shared experiences and meanings of our clients. Some of the more significant of these are explained in greater detail in Chapter 6. And this is not a simple matter of changing the therapists' levels of cultural sensitivity and competence to appreciate the cultures of their clients. The very ideology, philosophical bases, theory, body of knowledge and practice imperatives that speak to matters of culture at a broader level may not be as useful and enabling as we might want to believe. We may want to proceed deeper in our musings about client centred-ness, evidence and what constitutes best practice. Such consequences are the very bases for why new, culturally relevant knowledge, theory and practice norms are needed in occupational therapy[2].

The Western norm of contemporary occupational therapy – its form, meaning and functions – become inconceivable and misunderstood when applied in non-Western social contexts. More than half of the world's population is situated outside of the (Western) social contexts that gave rise to occupational therapy's raison d'être. Tacit social norms of independence, autonomy, self-efficacy and unilateral determination brought to bear on a clientele that prefers collective identity over individual identity, interdependence over autonomy, and hierarchy over equality, can produce some difficulties or might even be disastrous to people's sense of health and well-being. Like a square peg being forced into a round hole, the resulting incongruence can achieve the opposite of the enabling and empowering promises of occupational therapy. This can be reminiscent of certain colonial attitudes from a bygone era in which the information and assistance being prescribed from the dominant culture to *the other* results in superficial compliance to form and procedure, yet deficient in profound meaning, enabling and empowering.

Occupational Therapy As Culture

The critical examination of fit between occupational therapy's meanings and its clients' world of meanings is treated in this book as a profound matter of culture. When culture is viewed from such a perspective that transcends matters of individual attribute and embodiment, then culture is permitted to take into account the broader social processes, outside of the self in the social realm, that manufacture the categories of distinction into which such individual attributes become located. Your view from this regard will necessarily require you to proceed beyond cultural sensitivity at the individual level, towards a curiosity for the cultural construction of the profession and practice of occupational therapy itself. Examine this construal of culture closely and you may notice that occupational therapy, as a profession, possesses within it all of the features that would qualify it as a cultural entity. Occupational therapy has, for example, a shared specialised language[3], common learned values, and certain tacit and expressed rules of conduct, common social practices, and a developing body of profession-centred knowledge. A visit to almost any occupational therapy practice settings will reveal many of its cultural *artefacts*. By artefacts, we not only include material objects like splints, orthoses, long-handled reachers, etc., but also what occupational therapists regard to be worth knowing and doing. Conceptual models, theory and the assessment tools, new and evolving concepts like occupational deprivation[4] and occupational justice[5] represent some of occupational therapy's cultural artefacts.

More Than Individuals, Race and Ethnicity

So while the conventional treatment of culture in occupational therapy has been advanced along the lines of race and ethnicity, discoursed as individual markers of distinction – of therapists and clients – there is a need to expand its scope and definition to include social processes, of which the profession of occupational therapy as we know it qualifies. By recognising professional systems like occupational therapy or medicine as cultural entities, we are afforded a more useful framework for making sense of culture as a fundamental consideration in the construction of and treatment of meaning in the daily (occupational) lives of the patient-client. To be unaware of the essential cultural nature of occupation and occupational therapy is to be ignorant of a large portion of a comprehensive and just understanding of meaning in the lives of the populations we endeavour to serve. Discoursing occupational therapy as a cultural system in its own right steers us away from maintaining a perspective of culture in our profession as one in which the client is viewed and appreciated as an embodiment of static, stereotypical attributes.

This shift in defining and regarding culture holds important implications for this profession. As the emphasis in the culture discourse shifts from individual to profession, matters of inclusion and equity need to be critically revisited. Instead of seeing the problems of cultural relativism as existing at the individual level, the profession and all that it subsumes – its ideology, philosophy, epistemology, theory and practice forms – are brought into this spotlight of scrutiny. Congruent with the maxim, we can never be separate from the things we create and hold to be true, it can now be averred that the core concepts, ideology, knowledge and practice forms of contemporary occupational therapy are the manufactures of people who are situated in a particular sphere of shared experiences and views of 'normal'. Occupational therapy is culture-bound.

Culturally Out of Sync With Society?

Occupational therapy is truly powerful when its practice and the ideas that inform and guide it are congruent in spirit, truth and meaning to the client's worlds of the same. Occupational therapy's processes and benefits must resonate directly and meaningfully to the client's real world of home and community. Until now, we have not really asked the crucial and diffi-cult questions of relevance of our profession to and with the communities we serve. We have regarded and maintained our discourse to be universally true and applicable without having broached the difficult and necessary questions like: 'Does occupational therapy actually matter and is it as valuable and meaningful as we had been taught it to be?' And yet, despite the tacit understanding that occupational therapy does matter, occupational therapists find themselves still having to explain to their clients, to their fellow health team colleagues, and to the public, what they think occupational therapy is.

If we take a moment to explore how occupational therapists define and talk about 'occupation' through our own literature, textbooks, educational programme websites and then ask people – be they relatives, friends and clients – how they define or explain what the word occupation means, it does not take long to realise that we may not all be conversing on the same cultural page. We all hold differing understandings of 'occupation' created within different spheres of experience. When consulting several English language dictionaries for the definition of occupation, it may be difficult to find definitions that adequately capture the constellation of meanings occupational therapists ascribe to 'occupation'. Comparing and contrasting the varying definitions of the core concept of the profession of occupational therapy may reveal a disconnection between what occupational therapists mean by *occupation* and what their clients understand it to be.

Reconceptualising Occupation

岩

Situating Occupational Therapy's Knowledge
Why Alternative Conceptualisations and Models of Occupational Therapy Are Required

Occupational scientists[6] have invested much into the essentiality of occupation as a determinant in people's health and well-being. The establishment of this emerging academic discipline may hinge on the veracity of this dualism. The link between occupation and well-being, though it might resonate strongly among many who abide in Western social norms, has yet to be adequately validated – particularly for those who are culturally situated outside of the existential, individual-centred, rational and reflective Western world. The growth of occupational science might be challenged by the universalistic underpinnings of its research[7] mandates. There may be a need for a more fundamental discussion, particularly involving culture as a fundamental determinant in the meanings people ascribe to doing and agency. And we may need to determine whether human beings truly are reflective occupational beings, particularly when the construct of occupation, in the context of how occupational scientists and occupational therapists discourse it, does not exist in many of the Eastern and aboriginal lexicons around the world. Hence, in this book, reconceptualising occupation for those who live outside of Western cultural norms is purposely advanced.

Throughout this book, culture will be defined as: 'shared experiences and common spheres of meaning', and the (collective) social processes by which distinctions, meanings, categorisations of objects and phenomena are created and maintained. Rather than culture's usual reduction to individual matters like race and ethnicity, demonstrated in the segregation and labelling of people into categorical groupings according to certain static and stereotypically individualised features, culture will be discoursed as a particular concept as well as a dynamic process. Culture will represent both the common markers of distinction that people ascribe to categories of objects and phenomena, as well as to the dynamic process by which these distinctions and categories are created, maintained and transmitted.

Conventional Views of Culture in Occupational Therapy

From this particular perspective, there is awareness that culture is also *cultural*. That is to say, the meanings of culture, too, are not universal but constructed according to the varying spheres of shared experience from which the distinction is being made. In other words, culture means something different to people according to the varying shared understandings bounded by place and time that form the point of reference from which culture is being defined and understood. As stated earlier, popular notions of culture today in the industrialised world appear to refer to aspects of race and ethnicity so that a person's culture might be ascribed according to his or her country of origin or skin colour and physical features. This means that the meaning of culture is not limited to static markers of distinction of individual embodiments, and that these distinctions are created by and agreed upon by people who share a particular common context.

These views of culture – constructed as static individual attributions – are problematic on several levels. Readers examining their own occupational therapy practices may find that many clients do not fit neatly into the stereotypical patterns and categorisations attributed to language, physical features, behaviour patterns, etc., that are associated with their labelled 'culture'. Your client may possess an Indian surname and have all of the physical characteristics of a person originating from South Asia but may speak English with a cockney accent, prefer to eat Schezchuan food, and groove to the sounds of hip hop and American R&B. Applying individual-centred strategies of cultural sensitivity competently in an increasingly global and post-modern practice context can seem futile and even inappropriate at times. And applying an occupational therapy theoretical framework based on middle-American[8] culture may be ineffective, perhaps even inequitable, to many of our clients.

Despite our persistence to treat culture as a static set of features abiding within the individual, there is a growing awareness that culture is just as much about a dynamic social phenomenon that changes depending on location and time. Western views of culture have coincided with certain *rational*[9] views of the world. This would be the tendency to make sense of the world and its matter through the study of its parts (which are ultimately believed to be logically and systematically reducible from complex wholes). There is a corresponding tendency to view nature and the cosmos, including animate and inanimate objects as definable, divisible and therefore understandable. Westerners have demonstrated a historical tendency to group and categorise what they see, as if the whole can be understood by studying its finite parts.

However, the categorisation process does not stop there. Behind the propensity to separate elements and phenomena in the world into distinct parts and to categorise them is the tendency to classify these categories or distinctions into some kind of ranking order. Usually, the categories and the valuation of these groupings are enacted by the beholder who assumes a position of privilege and power. This is usually unwittingly carried out in the seemingly benign process of describing *the other* in relation to one's own position or privileged situation. It is evident whenever one's own standards or views of 'normal' are applied to evaluate and explain the objects and phenomena of *other* people situated in a different context. By which or by whose arbitrary standards did people of the non-Western world find themselves pejoratively and subordinately described as 'primitive', unclean, savage, and in need of cultivation? How did humans get to be more valued than other animals or elements of what we refer to as nature? Smith[3] and others have highlighted examples of this practice by pointing to the traditional lay-out of most

Situating Occupational Therapy's Knowledge
Why Alternative Conceptualisations and Models of Occupational Therapy Are Required

Victorian era museums of natural history. A walk through such a museum would typically lead you through a rational progression of lower forms of life to the highest (*Homo sapiens*). The ability to reason and engage in rational thinking might be at the top of the criteria employed to make these distinctions and rankings. There may even be a further categorisation and ranking of *Homo sapiens* as a species in which the 'ascent of man' is predicated on the development and use of tools. Placing and maintaining rational man in a privileged position at the top of his own arbitrarily devised classification system appears to be in operation today. Stone axes and wooden implements have been replaced by sophisticated weapons of war and efficient means for generating material profits in a global economy. If rational thought and action are the criteria for competence, then modern research and biomedicine would play an instrumental role in reifying this arbitrary ranking of human potential.

These perspectives on culture still persist today in the Western world, and are also evident in varying forms in Western occupational therapy, wherever there is need, albeit with good intentions, to *cultivate* the *other*. We should stop and ask ourselves: to whose cultural standards and norms are we trying to cultivate our clients to attain? Are the ideals of autonomy, independence, self-efficacy, unilateral control over nature and circumstances that we take for granted as being right in Western occupational therapy truly helpful, adaptive and enabling for those who abide in a different value pattern and norms of daily living?

The notion that *Homo sapiens* ought to cultivate themselves and others to some higher level of existence – or at least to the lifestyle patterns shared by those of the dominant culture – is amply visible historically in the world at large as well as in the world of occupational therapy. The colonial conquest of so-called inferior and primitive peoples by technologically and militarily advanced Northern/Westerns nations, of Southern and Eastern nations, were often explained and justified as the need to cultivate or emancipate the other. It is unfortunate that the term 'occupation', though we would like to use it in a very different regard, carries a historical construal of this very dynamic. What we may need to keep in mind as our profession discourses the social vision of occupation, as seen in new concepts like *occupational deprivation*[4], *occupational justice*[5] or *occupational apartheid*[10], is the Western-centric, existential bias that we unwittingly bring into our practices. The cultural element that is embedded in such philosophical and ideological development is borne in the question: what qualifies these ideas as particularly helpful and just? Whose cultural standards of what is good, beautiful and right are being applied to whose experiences and circumstances of reality? What qualifies a piece of artwork as beautiful or worthless, or an approach or idea in occupational therapy as being adaptive and right is debatable and will differ according to the particular perspectives and value patterns of the beholder or person(s) making the assessment. What these assertions underscore is the requirement to pay greater attention to culture and the manifestations of a particular (dominant) world view as assessments of those who abide in a different world view and sphere of experiences are being manufactured. For the occupational therapist, this means paying greater attention to respecting and ceding more credence to the client's views of reality.

A Matter of Perspective

If cultural forms and artefacts represent certain markers of distinction, then often the mundane and 'normal' in the reference culture remains invisible and unremarkable. It seems paradoxical that people situated in one sphere of experiences, say in Western Europe, might find the mundane and normal practices of people residing in East Asia remarkable. The daily routine for many Asians of eating a bowl of rice with two slender sticks might be seen as unusual and if this were not the 21st century, perhaps would require 'cultivation' to the more civilised practice of eating meat and potatoes on a plate with a knife and fork. The practice of studying and making sense of the other, with the sense that the other should be ultimately cultivated to emulate the practice patterns of the reference culture, was pervasive in the social sciences up to a few decades ago. Anthropological studies of the other – of naked, 'filthy', dark skinned people in grass skirts living 'primitively' in mud huts – were abundant. These depictions of the other were amusing ('thank God we're so lucky and don't have to live in squalor like that'), often carried unspoken sensations of superiority and a patronising view to want to 'save' them from themselves. All too often, the samples were studied and forgotten as the researchers endeavoured to find other 'amusing' and remarkable people and their lifestyles to discover. Social scientific journals from the 1950s and 1960s chronicle how scientists, situated in a Western sphere of experiences, depicted the other according to their own culturally bound understandings of normal.

Unfortunately, vestiges of this particular treatment of culture are pervasive in occupational therapy today. By treating culture as an individual attribute and being largely blind to the mundane and normal in the reference culture, Western occupational therapy scholars and practitioners have maintained to a large extent, the (Western) cultural boundaries of occupational therapy, its exclusive production of knowledge and the translation of its ideology and philosophy to practice.

Occupational Therapy's Grand Narrative as Culturally Bound

Students, practitioners, researchers and educators of occupational therapy, acculturated into North American life in particular, have had the good fortune of encountering the form, meaning and function of occupational therapy that is more familiar to their own contexts of day-to-day experience. North American occupational therapists have had the advantage of studying the ideas and theory of occupational therapy that fit better with their own cultural view of the world. Unfortunately, it does not stop there, for our assumptions about the nature of human agency, its components, organisation and meanings, appear to be imbued with universal qualities which transcend cultural boundaries and seem resistant to attempts at refuting or altering them. After all, what could possibly be wrong with a therapeutic approach driven by an ideology that seeks to empower individuals to improve or actualise themselves through rational, purposeful action? Few Westerners would take issue with a profession that seeks to assist people to *be* and *become*[11], through the use of one's *hands energised by mind and will*[12]. The ideals of a distinct agent self, celebrating autonomy, self-reliance, unilateral control of a separate, distinct, environment and circumstance, are familiar hallmarks of contemporary occupational therapy knowledge and theory. These ideals resonate so fundamentally with American value patterns and world views that few would question this narrative. Some of these ideals seem so morally 'right' and agree with the ethical practices of the dominant culture from which they have emerged that perhaps the entire world ought to have them as well.

The Need for Alternative, Culturally Relevant Theoretical Frameworks

In our clinical practices, we gain glimpses of this fundamental issue of incongruent narratives when clients have difficulty complying with *our* best intentions to assist them. Whether it is the elderly man who wonders why he is being encouraged to perform daily living tasks independently despite his family's insistence to do most of it for him, or a young aboriginal woman who consistently shows up in the afternoon for her scheduled mid-morning OT sessions (much to the staff's consternation), there is a tendency to construct such phenomena as a problem situated in the client or at the nexus between client and therapist, rather than to some set of philosophical or (cultural) value patterns embedded in the ideology or the structure of the therapy itself. If not deduced to be a language or communication issue, it might be understood as a problem with the client's particular *culture* that has fallen short of the requirements of occupational therapy. We might even draw the pejorative conclusion that the client is 'difficult' or 'non-compliant', thinking it incredulous that anyone might be at odds with the rightness of the therapeutic process or the ideology that drives it. Rarely, do we question the possibility that the problem might actually sit within occupational therapy itself and the cultural elements embedded in its perspectives on truth and normalcy, and frameworks that explain and guide its interventions.

The implications and consequences of implementing therapeutic interventions that are out of sync with local people's realities and shared meanings are profoundly important. They need paying attention to. Delivering an occupational therapy that is out of cultural context could result in a health service that therapists and clients have difficulties comprehending and therefore rob the profession of its meaning and potential to contribute something positive and truly useful to society. At worst, occupational therapy could be an agent of oppression, colonising and perhaps further marginalising people by requiring them to acquire competencies that are maladaptive and run counter to their basic value patterns[2].

In this book, the supporting ideologies underpinning occupational therapy, for example the assumption that humans are *occupational beings*, construed as cross-cultural universals are questioned and challenged. In order to bring an occupational therapy that is equitable, beneficial and culturally safe[13,14] into the lives of *other* peoples, whether they are geographically located in the Northern or Southern hemisphere, culture in occupational therapy needs to be understood on its own terms from the *other*'s vantage. It follows then that culture needs to be a fundamental consideration in the structure and content of occupational therapy epistemology, theory and practice.

REFERENCES

[1] Iwama M. The kawa (river) model: nature, life flow & the power of culturally relevant occupational therapy. In: Kronenberg F, Algado SA, Pollard N. (eds), Occupational Therapy Without Borders – Learning from the Spirit of Survivors, Edinburgh: Churchill Livingstone; 2005

[2] Iwama M. The issue is … toward culturally relevant epistemologies in occupational therapy. American Journal of Occupational Therapy 2003; 57(5):582–588

[3] Smith MJ. Culture: Reinventing the Social Sciences. Buckingham: Open University Press; 2000

[4] Whiteford G. Occupational deprivation: global challenge in the new millennium. British Journal of Occupational Therapy 2000; 64(5):200–210

[5] Townsend E, Wilcock AA. Occupational justice and client-centred practice: a dialogue-in-progress. Canadian Journal of Occupational Therapy 2004; 71(2):75–87

[6] Clark F. Occupational embedded in real life: inter-weaving occupational science and occupational therapy, 1993 Eleanor Clarke Slagle lecture. American Journal of Occupational Therapy 1993; 44:1067–1078

[7] Iwama MK. Editorial: revisiting culture in occupational therapy: a meaningful endeavor. OTJR: occupation, participation and health 2004; 24(1):2–3

[8] Gans H. Middle American Individualism. New York: The Free Press; 1988

[9] Iwama M. Meaning and inclusion: revisiting culture in occupational therapy. Australian Occupational Therapy Journal 2004; 51(1):1–2

[10] Kronenberg F, Pollard N. Overcoming occupational apartheid: a preliminary exploration of the political nature of occupational therapy. In: Kronenberg F, Algado SA, Pollard N. (eds), Occupational Therapy Without Borders – Learning from the Spirit of Survivors. Edinburgh: Churchill Livingstone; 2005

[11] Wilcock A. Reflections on doing, being, and becoming. Canadian Journal of Occupational Therapy 1998; 65:248–256

[12] Reilly M. Occupational therapy can be one of the great ideas of 20th century medicine. American Journal of Occupational Therapy 1962; 16:1–9

[13] Ramsden I. *Kawa whakaruruhau* – cultural safety in nursing education in Aotearoa: report to the Ministry of Education. Wellington: Ministry of Education; 1990

[14] Jungerson K. Culture, theory and the practice of occupational therapy in New Zealand/Aotearoa. American Journal of Occupational Therapy 1992; 46:745–750.

CHAPTER 2

Cross-Cultural Concepts As the Building Blocks of Conceptual Models

Occupation

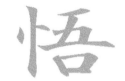

悟

Cross-Cultural Concepts As the Building Blocks of Conceptual Model

In the first chapter a broader definition and treatment of culture was introduced with some inferences drawn about its fundamental bearing on the production of knowledge, theory and practice in contemporary occupational therapy. Progressing beyond culture's usual treatment as a static mark or individual emblem of distinction (like race or ethnicity), culture was also discussed as a dynamic process by which such individual distinctions and the categories that function to delineate and organise such distinctions are socially manufactured (or *constructed*[1,2]). Collective agreement on the meaning of shared social experiences was speculated to be the important basis by which meanings were ascribed to phenomena and objects we experience and perceive in our world. It follows then, that rather than a single universal truth or set of authoritative understandings to explain phenomena and objects in the world for all people, there is in reality, a rich diversity in world views and interpretations of truth contingent on diverse spheres of shared experiences. The implications of this broader way of understanding culture for occupational therapy are significant and far-reaching. In terms of theory, the spectre of a large developing body of theoretical models that carry assumptions of universal application are now brought into question, scrutinised for cultural relevancy and cultural safety[3]. This broader definition of culture also draws occupational therapists to question whether our current epistemology[4] qualifies as 'worth knowing' for people who purportedly abide in a different understanding of reality. In occupational therapy, the need for alternative, culturally relevant theoretical material was raised due to exclusionary consequences that might occur when narratives of truth and doing, created and situated in one particular social context, are applied out of original context into another.

Occupational therapists are educated to regard theory (including conceptual models) as useful frameworks that can function to describe, explain, validate[5] and guide[6] occupational therapy. And when such theories are considered valid, they may also be utilised by therapists to predict[7] practice outcomes. Without theoretical material to guide our interventions and provide plausible rationale for occupational therapy, Krefting[8] suggested that, practice would amount to little more than a process of 'trial and error'. But theoretical frameworks can also do more than guide the practice of occupational therapy. Having useful, credible models to explain human occupation, occupational performance and the processes of occupational therapy can help define the profession, demonstrate our philosophy and even clarify and strengthen our professional identity.

The favourable impact that theory and conceptual models have had on the profession of occupational therapy over the past three decades is undeniable. Theoretical material, such as the Canadian model of occupational performance[9] (CMOP), the model of human occupation[10] (MOHO), as well as Reed and Sanderson's concepts of occupational therapy[11] and Reilly's occupational behaviour paradigm[12] that preceded them, have helped to delineate occupational therapy from medicine, define the profession, and lead it through a renaissance[13] of occupation.

While contemporary occupational therapy theory commands an essential place and role in this profession, the utility, meaning and the universal applicability of these materials warrant attention. In particular, occupational therapists may need to examine critically whether their theory retains its relevance to its entire clientele – even those clients situated in other contexts. As occupational therapists attend to the growing diversity of needs of people representing life circumstances and conditions foreign to the very social contexts that informed the construction of their existing theory and approaches, they may need to consider new and alternate theoretical materials to bring occupational therapy's mandates into better agreement with varying world views and ways of knowing. Are the explanations of occupation and well-being in our current models that were constructed in Western social contexts applicable to clients abiding in a different cultural reality?

In this chapter, the core concept of occupational therapy is examined with particular consideration given to its cross-cultural utility in light of the meanings ascribed to it within the profession. Meanings of doing reflected to one's own existence appears to be a tacit value in many Western views of reality. 'If I can't do what I want to do, then there's no point in living', may not be such a peculiar utterance in Western social life. In an egalitarian value structure, individual agency can take on an essentiality that supersedes all other basic requirements. While Western occupational therapy theorists have enjoyed the privilege of being able to tie their conceptions of occupation to something regarded to be essential to life and existence in the context of Western spheres of experience and meaning, others located in alternate spheres of daily experience may not be able to relate to it in the same way nor understand the power and promise of occupational therapy that Westerners proclaim it to offer.

Occupation as a Cross-Cultural Construct

How do the complex meanings and essential ties to human well-being ascribed to the concept of occupation by occupational therapists situated in the West fare when taken into *other* cultural contexts? Do they carry the same veracity and explanatory power when placed in alternate spheres of social experience? Before developing and advancing their theory and knowledge systems, occupational therapists urgently need to examine whether the meanings that have been attributed to the experience of human agency really are as universally powerful to explain occupation's appropriateness and benefit for all. While there are many who may question the need to examine critically the fundamental tenets of our profession – like the meaning of occupation and the basic premises of fulfilment and well-being that are associated with it – others (many of whom comprise our own clients and professional colleagues) may point out that these same assumptions and tenets do not resonate similarly in their lives. At times, these ideas are experienced as if they were cast in some unfamiliar context of meanings. If such incongruities do exist and there is a will for our membership to direct this profession towards a culturally inclusive and meaningful service for all, the ideology, knowledge, theories and practice of occupation need to be re-examined and possibly reconsidered.

Understanding the cross-cultural utility of occupation, as occupational therapists have discoursed it, holds profound implications for the current practice, research and the future outlook for this profession. In this chapter, *occupation's* intimate ties to the social and cultural contexts in which it had been constructed and given its meanings is examined and a bold, possibly audacious, imperative is put forward; occupation needs to be reconceptua-lised, drawing its meanings from and anchoring its definitions to the cultural contexts in which it is to be applied. This critical analysis of occupation is propagated through a comparative juxtaposition of social and cultural conditions to illustrate its cross-cultural implications. By doing this, occu-pational therapists are enabled to appreciate further the profound significance of culture. How occupational therapists the world over regard and conceptua-lise occupation in different social and cultural contexts will determine to a large extent how durable and universal our profession's core concept is and whether there should be some leeway given to reconceptualise occupation to resonate in other cultural situations. Reconceptualising occupation and allowing the concept to be anchored to what people in varying cultural contexts hold to be essential to their lives may determine how meaningful and inclusive the idea of occupational therapy can be for all.

Culture, Context and the Ascription of Meaning

Culture forms the basis to this context-situated examination of occupation. In the previous chapter, the familiar constructions of culture were expanded to include the process by which meanings were ascribed to objects and phenomena according to common spheres of social experience. These spheres of experience were explained to be situated in time and place, thus presenting culture as a dynamic as much as it was the marks of distinction ascribed to people. Stated in another way, culture is 'a complex interplay of shared meanings that represent and shape the individual and collective lives of people'. This viewpoint of culture is consistent with what is referred to often in the post-modern genre of social science discourse as a position of cultural relativism. Briefly, unlike the universalism associated with views and constructions of truth in the modernist era, cultural relativists would take the view that truth is relative to each individual within their environment, based upon the prevailing discourse of his or her society[14]. By environment, the social context is of primary concern. This viewpoint of culture is also consistent with social constructionism[1,2]. It is consistent with Berger and Luckmann's[15] treatise on the sociology of knowledge, that humans socially construct their realities. Such a view is radical when taken as a significant departure from rejection of the line of epistemology handed down to us through the enlightenment thinkers that essentially regarded truth as singularly universal (and therefore not variable according to social context), separate to the knower, and knowable through persistence and systematic (scientific) enquiry[4].

When such a powerful system of explanation has pervaded virtually all aspects of currently accepted knowledge production in the health professions, even within occupational therapy, alternative experiences and different but equally valid constructions of reality and truth can often be overlooked or even dismissed. The cultures and societies of Asia, for example, which make up more than half[16] of the world's population, have their own systems and traditions of ethics, religion, politics, and aesthetics, forged over millennia that diverge substantially from the social contexts that supported the enlightenment of 18th century Europe. To accept that such aberrations of epistemology and ontology exist depending on different spheres of experience and place requires occupational therapists to rethink the veracity and universal applicability of their current constructions of truth, including the universality of the concept of occupation and the meanings of occupational therapy. This reconsideration of the profession's core ideas is a necessary first step towards making our theory, epistemology and practice culturally inclusive[4].

Culturally relevant occupational therapy is a challenging position to consider for obvious reasons. Rather than an intention to cultivate the other to our own cultural constructions of reality, we may need to consider cultivating occupational therapy and its current ideology to suit our clients' diverse worlds of meanings.

Universal Versus Particular Understanding of Objects and Phenomena

Culture is much more than a trait or a feature embodied in the identities of ourselves and our clients. It also represents a social process by which our shared experiences and interpretations of truth (and therefore our values and valuing of objects and phenomena around us) support ascription and associations of meaning within occupational therapy.

Christmas Across Cultural Frontiers

To illustrate this point an example, quite distanced from matters usually associated with occupational therapy, is offered utilising the culturally situated understandings of the Christian holiday of Christmas. To the Westerner who subscribes to Christian ideals, there is a familiar religious meaning to December 25. It is the day to commemorate the birth of Jesus Christ who is believed, by those who share the experience of being Christians, to be both God and Saviour of the world. It is a day that symbolises hope for those who share such meanings and evokes feelings of joy and celebration, and the urge to perform deeds of goodwill. Hence gifts are exchanged on Christmas Day. There are variations in the rituals and traditions associated with Christmas, which have developed over historical and social contexts. Some exchange gifts on Christmas Eve, whereas others situated in other locations might leave their gifts and presents for loved ones under a decorated tree, to be opened on Christmas Day. The rituals and forms may differ, but the deeper and ultimate meanings that support these occupations, can be reflected back to, at least for devout Christians, the original meaning and celebration of Christ's birth.

Christmas also exists in Japan, but the original meanings of Christmas there were informed by a very different historical and social context. In Japanese contexts, Christmas is hardly about celebrating the birth of Jesus Christ. Now it is fair to say that cultural changes continue to occur within the Western world, and that the perception and meaning of Christmas has also changed and diversified. However, the association of Christmas as a Christian event, marked in importance by national holidays, persists.

For the majority of Japanese who are not practising Christians, it is about *Santa Ojisan* (uncle Santa) bringing gifts to children, special sale campaigns in the shopping malls and department stores and a boon for any commercial enterprise that can profit from this imported Western reason for making merry. In Japanese cities like Tokyo and Osaka, since at least the early 1980s, it can be difficult to reserve a night's rest in a major hotel on Christmas Eve. Most of the available rooms are booked well in advance by romantic couples who are eager to carry out what seems to have become a popular ritual associated with Christmas Eve and Christmas Day. On December 24, each partner will dress in attractive, fashionable attire and have dinner in the hotel's fine restaurant. The hoteliers, who are well attuned to the auspiciousness of the date have planned special multiple course dinner sets befitting the occasion. Some of the dinner plans are tied together with the room reservation. During the dinner date, the couple will exchange 'x'mas gifts'. Later on, the couple will spend a night together in the hotel. Besides the hotel Christmas experience, Japanese parents may give gifts to their young children, or a family might share a special cake on this occasion.

Some of the traditional forms and rituals associated with and practised around Christmas in Western countries have been adopted and appreciated in a different way by many Japanese, but the profound religious symbolic meaning associated with it in Western spheres of experiences remain remarkable. The dates and rituals may be similar but there are different spheres of experience associated with it that contribute to its respective meanings. The form on the surface may look similar but the underlying value and meanings ascribed to it can differ remarkably. A North American Christian visitor journeying to Japan during his Christmas holidays might observe the Japanese treatment of Christmas and feel offended by it. He may strongly feel the need to cultivate Japanese constructions of Christmas to enable them to appreciate the occasion in *the proper* way.

Instead of an occasion like Christmas that acquires certain meanings from the surrounding social context, we might now consider another matter closer to the subject of occupational therapy. What happens to a concept like occupation when we view it in various contexts of culture? If we were to insert a social phenomenon, such as 'human action' into a similar comparison between two different shared social spheres of experience, a similar contrast of associated meanings as what was demonstrated with the concept of Christmas would be apparent.

Occupation enters new social frontiers already imbued richly with culturally situated meanings. There is very little critical analysis of the cultural qualities of occupation on either side of the export/import continuum. Current definitions of occupations demonstrate a valuing that is particularly reflective of Western experience and world views. To an East Asian importer of occupational therapy – a person who has constructed their perceptions and views of the world through a different set of traditions, religious and philosophical tenets, beliefs of what is true, worth knowing and worth doing – the social context that has emerged our current definitions of occupation look particularly individual-centred and rational. Such a world view appears to construct self and nature as separate, discrete entities that reflect a kind of divinely set order. It appears to be an order that has placed the individual self in a superior relation to nature, in which the latter and its circumstances are relegated to be exploited and managed.

Is the construction or definition of occupational therapy's core concept truly challenging and problematic to others? A large part of the answer, from a social constructionist perspective, is found in and explained by differences in the social contexts that support the specific meanings attributed to the concept of meaningful human action, or 'human occupation'. The concept of occupation with its rich associated meanings, never did exist in similar social frames nor in the lexicons of many non-Western nations and cultural groups. Japanese occupational therapists have struggled for decades to translate occupation into their own language and social contexts of understanding. The Japanese, through much deliberation resigned themselves to use the term *sagyou* – a word approximating tedious, laborious work in English (Figure 2.1). Though the same system of written characters are used in the various dialects of Chinese, occupational therapists in China, Hong Kong, Taiwan, and Singapore, for example, use different characters/symbols or words for 'occupational therapy'[17].

作業　療法

Sagyou　　　　　　　　　　　　　Ryouhou

Figure 2.1 Translation of 'occupational therapy' into Japanese using Chinese characters. *Sagyou* can be roughly translated as work of the tedious and laborious kind, while *ryouhou* is the common Japanese interpretation for 'therapy'.

The problem is not simply one of language in which the other merely needs to find better words to represent an *occupation* that is believed to exist universally despite issues of varying contexts and spheres of experiences. Rather, it may be that specific shared social contexts that give rise to the naming of objects and ascription of meaning to phenomena are unique to time and place. These social contexts, as a group, may not have valued meanings of individual actions identical to the modal Westerner's particular existential, rational and individual-oriented understandings ascribed to *occupation*.

Diverse Contexts of Occupational Therapy

A critical examination of the cross-cultural utility of occupational therapy's core construct has yet to penetrate the academic discourse in occupational therapy. It may not be a priority for many abiding within a dominant world view that assumes a singular truth and favours rational, universal explanations (a feature of grand theories) of phenomena to consider alternative world views and divergent spheres of human experience. There is not much value to such an exercise of critical reflection and subsequent action other than being benevolent to those *others* whose world views are situated outside of *normal*. On the other hand, alternative views of the world are often dismissed, treated as irrational, and judged to be simply 'wrong'. This would be an unfortunate attitude to maintain and disastrous for the profession of occupational therapy, for such indifference may mirror an attitude of intolerance towards diverse clients residing in Western contexts who hold world views, occupations and their meanings that abide outside of the dominant culture's boundaries of 'normal'.

It is paradoxical that the culture of science and its rationalistic procedures offer us glimpses of this potential problem. From an empirical vantage, issues of construct validity and generalisability of research outcomes to populations outside of those represented by the research sample (external validity) inform us that aberrations from certain norms can and do exist. Researchers, conscious of such threats to the reliability of a certain instrument or gathered data, go to extraordinary lengths to institute the required procedural rigour to minimise these effects of what can be described or attributed to the effects or consequences of *culture*.

Occupational therapists have much to gain from diverse world views and spheres of experience. An alternate cultural vantage provides the comparative foil that functions to raise the normally unremarkable to remarkable views and thereby expose the mundane and normal which would usually lay hidden in the tacit and shared assumptions situated within a particular cultural frame. Some readers may have been surprised to learn that what has always seemed normal to them, can look abnormal and extraordinary to others abiding in a different cultural experience of *normal*. When 'occupation' is viewed from an alternate cultural point of reference and interpretation of reality and meaning – one like Japan's, which has been frequently described in the social scientific literature as polytheistic[18], naturalistic[19], collectivist[20], interdependent[21], hierarchical in social structure[22], and temporally oriented to the present[23] – its universal relevance is questioned and placed in jeopardy. Few concepts are generalisable and relevant to entire populations. When concepts are generalised, the spectres of stereotyping and sweeping attributions of certain fixed characteristics to entire groups become possible.

Cultural Constructions of Self and Environment: Inadequacies of Dualisms

Embedded in and tacitly accepted as a given truth in contemporary views of occupation, as seen in our conceptual models raised out of Western world views, are the distinctions that separate the self and environment into two separate entities. These entities are not always perceived to be parallel or integrated. Rather, the structural relationship is one in which the self and environment are situated in opposition to each other. This perception crystallises in such analogies or metaphors that explain occupation as the bridge that connects the self to the environment. The emerging academic discipline of occupational science and the applied field of occupational therapy have a significant reliance on the veracity of this dualism. This is not an indictment on dualisms. Rather, the affinity for rational world views and the cultural capital that such views carry in occupational therapy is being made remarkable, for the purpose of recognising a point of dissonance in the theoretical and epistemological make-up of occupational therapy.

'Through our actions on the world around us, we occupy our environment, and in turn we derive a sense of being ...' could be an example statement that illustrates this dualism. A person from Japan, or an aboriginal group member, might have some difficulty grasping this explanation of occupation because the metaphor may not fit their own sensations of how they view the construction of 'self' in relation to the environment and others. By being acculturated and socialised into a different view of the cosmos – a pluralistic world view in which selves are inextricably integrated collectively with the environment – the suggestion that we occupy our environs through purposeful and meaningful action is amusing to consider but ultimately incredulous. 'Why do I have to exert any effort towards occupying something that I already occupy?'; 'The environment is an integrated part of me … how do I then occupy that?' may be the kind of questions asked in response to a typical rational explanation of occupation. In the realms of Eastern philosophies like Buddhism and ethical systems like Confucianism and Taoism, there is no strong sense of the centralised agent self or a separate and distinct environment to subjugate as one's own.

Also problematic to many non-Western people is the notion of mankind's stewardship[24] over, or utilitarian need to control, an environment or set of circumstances situated outside of, and placed in opposition to, the self[25]. Japanese people, as with other non-Western situated people may tend to hold a 'me in the world'[26] rather than 'me against the world' attitude that is consistent with subject–object dualisms. This may have a bearing on how the modal Japanese person may regard certain motivations for action in the world – especially pertaining to the perception, valuing and response to challenges encountered in daily living. Does one 'make a bee-line through the opposition' or 'break through barriers' rather than evade direct opposition or find some way to slip around those barriers like water around rocks and other obstacles in a river's flow? Can one accept or find a way to live with a particular circumstance or difficulty? The predominantly Euro-Western intellectual tradition of rationalism that separates, delineates and categorises the universe into separate discrete elements, handed down through the preceding centuries since at least the enlightenment era, has never been adequate to explain particular Japanese and Asian views of self, universe and the meaning of human being and existence. Neither would such knowledge adequately represent truth for aboriginal societies, nor any other social group outside of Euro-Western social experience, in the world.

Occupational therapists working with clients representing diverse cultures may have been perplexed, and perhaps frustrated by the difficulties incurred during the application of established occupational therapy theory or the measurement instruments supported by such theory. The culturally competent occupational therapist may need to add to their repertoire of skills, the ability to critically examine cultural assumptions of truth, morality, logic and individual agency embedded in and translated through their dominant theoretical materials, including conceptual models.

Decentralised 'Self', Collectivism and the Celebration of Dependence

The coincidence of a decentralised self and temporal orientation to the present, as features of Japanese shared experience, is worthy of some consideration when exploring the cultural boundaries of occupation. The positioning of self, the relative power ceded to collectives, appears to coincide with whether the past, present or future holds the greatest influence on one's world views. All three contribute to a context for the assembly and performance of human occupation in non-Western settings like Japan. When the spectre of rational, self-determinism is lessened and the tendency to reflect all matters to the solitary self loses much of its primacy, temporal orientation towards the future gives way to the consciousness of the here and now. In the Japanese experience, resignation of the future matters to *unme* or fate is a common practice. Collective will and collectively held future objectives appear to hold greater sway on guiding and influencing individual action. 'What I want to do' is strongly modified by the interests of the collective over any strong unilateral drive. The notion of 'becoming'[27] through 'doing' is typically perplexing to the modal Japanese person, whose sensation of personal agency and time are configured according to a different social context and structure from the one from which emerged the Western concept of occupation. 'What everyone in my social frame wants to do is what I want to do', is a particularly strong Japanese common feeling.

Amae: Normal Japanese Dependency As a Context for Human Agency

Other concepts or points of comparison pertaining to the Japanese social that are helpful in examining how occupation crosses cultural boundaries of meaning will be addressed more comprehensively in Chapters 4 and 5. The Japanese idea of *amae*[28] is introduced here as a final concept of comparison that further elucidates the cross-cultural viability of the Western-centric concept of occupation.

Amae is derived from the Japanese word for 'sweetness' and is a necessary, adaptive aspect of Japanese social relation. Though the construct of dependency in social relationships can be observed in most societies, social scientists specialising on Japan appear to have accepted the concept of *amae* into their interpretations and descriptions of dependent behaviour patterns in Japanese society[18,21]. What sets *amae* apart from so many other concepts used to describe the structure of the Japanese social, is that it is a Japanese concept and pervasively appears in virtually all aspects of Japanese social relations. Some scholars have gone so far as to regard *amae* as a unique form of dependence that sets Japanese society apart from other modern, industrial societies[20]. Doi articulated this behaviour pattern over 30 years ago in his publication titled 'Amae no Kouzou'[28] (the structure of dependence). Since then, *amae* as a concept has found its way into the lexicon of social scientific research in Japan and it seems that no comprehensive work concerning the Japanese *social* can forego mention of this popular concept.

Doi defines *amae* as: 'the need of an individual to be loved and cherished; the prerogative to presume and depend upon the benevolence of another' (p. 165). In this way, *amae* is seen to be both a noun (as a concept to describe a pattern of behaviour) and as a verb (to symbolise a behaviour – of seeking the indulgence of another). Doi likens *amae* to 'the craving of a new born child for close contact with its mother, and in the broader sense, the desire to deny the fact of separation that is an inevitable part of human existence, and to obliterate the pain that this separation involves' (p. 169). While the ideal of independence is pervasive in Western social life and serves as an important criterion in determining an individual's readiness to navigate their lives in the world and assert one's identity as separate from others, the opposite seems to be the norm in Japanese social experience. It may be thus unusual for the average Westerner to imagine that most Japanese, who regard *amae* to be a normal, natural emotion do not frustrate the 'drive to dependence' (p. 169) and will try to prolong it throughout their lives, even well into adulthood.

Japanese society, understood as vertically structured collectivism, affords much leeway for *amae* behaviour. In fact, it could be argued that life in modern Japan would be extremely difficult to navigate without demonstrating some aspect of *amae* behaviour or its associated language. *Amae*, or 'Japanese inter-dependency' holds fundamental bearing on how Japanese people construct meaning in human action. Not only are states of dependence tolerated, but actually expected as part of a pattern of normal, adaptive behaviour in Japanese social contexts of meaning. Every thing and every phenomenon is made sense of through the filter of human relationships in the Japanese brand of social relativism[29] and such relationships are configured in hierarchical structure held together by the glue of dependence and indulgence. This aspect of the Japanese social stands in direct opposition to the Western values of independence, self-efficacy and self-determinism that are so strongly and tacitly evident in occupational therapy theory. Collective agency supersedes individual agency. Before doing something that means something to me, doing something that holds meaning to the collective and is reasonable in the context of the dependence-indulgence structure of relationships, holds greater sway.

Though some limited descriptions of the Japanese social context, that contrast sharply in many instances with the spheres of experience in which the concept of occupation has been traditionally and conventionally enacted and inter-preted, have been employed to examine the cross-cultural viability of occu-pation, readers are encouraged to juxtapose their own cultural experiences to the grand narrative of occupational therapy. It is important not to limit your juxtapositions and comparisons to traditional interpretations of culture, along the lines of ethnicity, race or nationality. Socio-economic considerations, including spheres of experience around poverty; socio-political influences such as the case of people in former Eastern European countries transitioning from socialistic political states to capitalistic political states; the social contexts of urban situation and rural situation present some important and viable cultural points of reference. Shared spheres of experience around gender, sexual orientation, disenfranchisement, the institutions of modern medicine and institutions of higher learning, are some more examples of cultural situations that need to be considered in light of occupational therapy theory and epistemology. It is difficult to refute some casual observations that occupational therapy represents a culture and ideology based on middle-class, Western, female experience-oriented social norms and world views.

How the reader interprets the relativist and constructionist arguments put forward in these pages depends on one's particular take on reality and truth. If you regard truth to be singular, external to the self and universally applicable across cultural boundaries, then there will be little here to motivate you to alter and apply the mandate of occupational therapy to people situated outside of your social and cultural norms.

Much of the current discourse on culture in occupational therapy has centred on competency and sensitivity of practitioners towards clients and the cultural features and practices they are seen to embody, more than the cultural construction of occupational therapy itself, and the implications this holds when contemplating issues of meaning and inclusion in our clients' lives. Occupational therapists must now begin to enquire: with whose cultural norms do we view our clients, especially those clients who fall outside of our conceptions of the normal? Do our current epistemologies, ideologies, theories and practices in occupational therapy truly abide within the lived realities of those we serve? To what extent do occupational therapists situated outside of the mainstream social spheres of experience participate in our knowledge production and discourse? All of these questions represent formidable concerns for those who consume and contribute to the product contained in the pages of occupational therapy's professional literature and discourse. In our well-intentioned attempts to assist and perhaps cultivate the 'other' to our particular views of truth and reality, what we consider to be good, true and beautiful, often proceeds unquestioned and unaltered. This, despite such profound differences between our and their explanations of reality, truth, and what is worth knowing and what is worth doing.

The expressions of occupational therapy's theory, epistemology and practice norms have always been dominated by spheres of shared experience situated in the Western world. The current social construction of and ideology around occupation within occupational therapy discourse are readily appreciable in contemporary occupational therapy conceptual models as well as in the profession's mainstreams. As occupational therapy finds its way on the coat-tails of biomedicine into new international frontiers, all of these cultural artefacts of occupational therapy will inevitably run into cultural barriers, resulting in questions and challenges of meaning and utility from a position of cultural relevance. And occupational therapy should avail itself to these challenges, for a move towards cultural relevance and a more diverse discourse around the meaning of concepts and principles paying due respect to cultural context will advance occupational therapy in a more inclusive, relevant, powerful and equitable direction.

There is a subtle proclamation of power and authority in statements of ownership – of having propriety to a profession's history, traditions, epistemology and truth. That authoritative power is further canonised when coded into an exclusive set of concepts and language that favour a particular social and cultural context[30]. The challenge now stands for occupational therapy to acknowledge the exclusive leanings in theory and epistemology and to find and incorporate ways to expand its social vision; to make its enterprise truly relevant and equitable in the face of an increasingly diverse post-modern world. Occupational therapists and their clients located in contexts differing markedly from the West's have struggled to reconcile an alien lexicon, theoretical materials that reflect a different experience and appreciation of lived reality and a historical record that is interesting but ultimately someone else's. What we need are contributions of new theory and culturally relevant knowledge representative of the profession's broad and profoundly meaningful mandate. This also entails permitting the reconceptualisation of occupation to resonate on a basic level with people of diverse backgrounds. How occupational therapists regard cultural context for determining the meaning and power of occupation, will determine occupational therapy's utility and potential to meaningfully touch people's lives in truly useful ways. Only when this is adequately achieved will people close to us – our clients and our colleagues – cease to ask what occupation and occupational therapy mean.

REFERENCES

[1] Burr V. An Introduction to Social Constructionism. London: Routledge; 1995

[2] Gergen KJ. An Invitation to Social Construction. Thousand Oaks: Sage Publications; 1999

[3] Ramsden I. *Kawa whakaruruhau* – cultural safety in nursing education in Aotearoa: report to the Ministry of Education. Wellington: Ministry of Education; 1990

[4] Iwama M. The issue is … toward culturally relevant epistemologies in occupational therapy. American Journal of Occupational Therapy 2003; 57(5):582–588

[5] Clark PN. Theoretical frameworks in contemporary occupational therapy practice, Part 1. American Journal of Occupational Therapy 1979; 33:505–514

[6] Miller R. What is theory and why does it matter? In: Miller R, Sieg K, Ludwig F, Shortridge S, Van Deusen J. (eds), Six Perspectives on Theory for the Practice of Occupational Therapy. Rockville: Aspen Publishers Inc; 1988

7 Duldt B, Giffin K. Theoretical Perspectives for Nursing. Boston: Little, Brown & Co; 1985

8 Krefting L. The use of conceptual models in clinical practice. Canadian Journal of Occupational Therapy 1985; 52(4):173–178

9 Canadian Association of Occupational Therapists. Enabling Occupation: An Occupational Therapy Perspective. Toronto: CAOT Publications; 1997

10 Kielhofner GA. Model of Human Occupation: Theory and Application, 3rd edn. Baltimore: Williams and Wilkins; 2002

11 Reed K, Sanderson S. Concepts of Occupational Therapy. Baltimore: Williams and Wilkins; 1980

12 Van Deusen J. In: Miller R, Sieg K, Ludwig F, Shortridge S, Van Deusen J. Six Perspectives on Theory for the Practice of Occupational Therapy. Rockville: Aspen Publishers Inc; 1988

13 Whiteford G, Townsend E, Hocking C. Reflections on a renaissance of occupation. Canadian Journal of Occupational Therapy 2000; 67:61–69

14 Winch P. Understanding a primitive society. American Philosophical Quarterly 1964; 1(4):307–324

15 Berger P, Luckmann T. The Social Construction of Reality: A Treatise on the Sociology of Knowledge. Garden City, New York: Anchor Books; 1966

16 US Census Bureau. Report WP/98: world population profile, 1998. Washington, DC: US Government Printing Office; 1998

17 Sinclair K. Conference Proceedings: WFOT Presidential address. Third Asia Pacific Occupational Therapy Congress, Singapore. September 15–18; 2003

18 Johnson F. Dependency and Japanese Socialization: Psychoanalytic and Anthropological Investigations into Amae. New York: New York University Press; 1993

19 Lebra ST. Self in Japanese culture. In: Rosenberger NR. (ed.), Japanese Sense of Self. New York: Cambridge University Press; 1992

20 Hendry J. Understanding Japanese Society, 2nd edn. London: Routledge; 1987

21 Doi T. The Anatomy of Dependence. Tokyo, Japan: Kodansha International; 1973

22 Nakane C. Tate shakai no ningen kankei [Human relations in a vertical society]. Tokyo: Kodansha; 1970

23 Iwama M. A social perspective on the construction of occupational therapy in Japan. Unpublished doctoral dissertation. Takahashi: Kibi International University; 2001

24 Gustafson JM. Man and Nature: A Cross-Cultural Perspective. Bangkok: Chulalongkorn University Press; 1993

[25] Ellen RF The cognitive geometry of nature: A contextual approach. In: Descola P, Pálsson G. (eds), Nature and Society: Anthropological Perspectives. London: Routledge; 1996; 103–123

[26] Bellah R. Beyond Belief: Essays on Religion in a Post Traditional World. New York: Harper & Row; 1991

[27] Hasselkus B. The Meaning of Everyday Occupation. Thorofare, New Jersey: Slack Inc; 2002

[28] Doi T. Amae no kozo [The Anatomy of Dependence]. Tokyo: Kobundo; 1971 (in Japanese)

[29] Lebra S. Japanese Patterns of Behavior. Honolulu: University of Hawaii Press; 1976

[30] Iwama M. Occupation as a cross-cultural construct. In: Whiteford G, Wright-St Clair (eds), Occupation and Practice in Context. Sydney: Churchill Livingstone; 2004

Occupational Therapy Theory

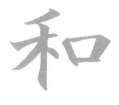

Cultural Inclusion and Exclusion

和

Viewed from a cultural relativist or constructionist perspective, few concepts, and the principles they combine to form, are accorded universal explanatory power. That is because concepts are constructed in and abide in specific cultural contexts of meaning which are situated in place and time. In the preceding chapter, the cross-cultural translation of occupation was briefly visited, drawing some attention to the potential problems that differences in meaning pose for the knowledge, theory and practice of occupational therapy. In this chapter an examination of the cultural construction of occupation continues but proceeds towards illuminating the cultural boundaries of contemporary occupational therapy through a brief but critical look at the profession's theory. Theory, which includes conceptual models, is the systematic representation of occupational therapy's grand narratives. They embody the profession's particular world views, values, social norms, viewpoints in relation to societal needs like disability and well-being. They articulate the language and concepts that are core to the profession, and even serve to guide and shape occupational therapy practice. Theory is of paramount importance to any health professional group. Without theory, occupational therapists would be no more than technicians delivering a service limited by recipes and procedural mandates set by others, rather than being led by comprehensive philosophical frameworks and specialised bodies of knowledge.

In this chapter, we examine the inextricable link between constructs (and the principles that bind them together in logical and meaningful ways) and the varying world views that subsume the situations or contexts that give rise to and support them. The same cultural concerns discussed in the first two chapters are maintained here. Do the narratives of shared experiences, views of truth and reality, and common meanings reflected in occupational therapy conceptual models agree with those of occupational therapists and their diverse clients? The philosophical basis to this particular critical view is based on the premise that we can never be fully separated from our ideas and that theories must be critically understood as extensions of the theorist's contextual world view.

If we continue with our broader understanding of culture, viewed simply as 'common spheres of experience' and includes both the markers and categories of distinction as well as the processes by which such distinctions are created, maintained and translated, then we need to examine the cultural nature of occupational therapy in a new and different way. Few occupational therapists situated in Western societies would take issue with the notion that the *occupation* in occupational therapy is defined as 'the domain of concern and the therapeutic medium of occupational therapy'[1]. 'Occupation is explained to be everything that people do to occupy themselves, and can include groups of activities and tasks of everyday life, named, organized, and given value and meaning by individuals and a culture'[1]. Culture in this statement is treated as a secondary or tertiary concern. However, in the realm of Western spheres of experience in occupational therapy, occupation appears to be imbued with more profound meanings. Meanings that go as far as defining the construction of one's 'self' become essential to a society that places fundamental emphasis on the individual as a reflective, rationally minded, independent entity. The construct of 'occupation' subsumes many of the common assumptions that many Westerners hold to be true of their world and how being and individual identity are inextricably tied to what we 'do'. Christiansen viewed 'occupation as the principal means through which people develop and express their personal identities'[2]. He added that: 'competence in performance of tasks and occupations contributes to identity shaping and that the realization of an acceptable identity contributes to coherence and well-being'[2]. For theory, Christiansen drew primarily from Mead's[3] work on *symbolic interactionism*, and from Piaget[4] – that even infants come to know the world through the action of 'doing'. Within similar shared societal contexts bounded by time and place, the explanations for occupation resonate plausibly and are reified through agreement and reinforcement among those who share that particular perspective of truth. They remain uncontested for a period for there is little priority or urgency to question that which is tacitly accepted as true.

The cultural construction of *occupation* in occupational therapy is supported by basic streams of modern social thought and social theory, particularly involving, but not limited to, the concepts of *agency, praxis* and *reflexivity*. That the core tenets of occupational therapy often abide within explanations offered by modern social scientists has helped to reify it, at least in the West. With such tacit perspectives towards self, society and the environs, it may be difficult for Western people to imagine *occupation* to hold *particular*, culture-bound meanings, shaped and influenced by prevailing social and cultural contexts.

Celebrated notions of 'self' and identity have come to inhabit our ideas of wellness and healthy states of being in occupational therapy. Wilcock[5] has coined what has arguably become the defining slogan for occupational therapists: 'doing, being, and becoming'. Westerners would probably agree that fundamental elements of our *beings* and what we aspire to become are primarily shaped and determined by what we *do*. Suffering insult to one's ability to 'do', due to some unfortunate event or circumstance, represents an essential problem and appropriate rationale for occupational therapy intervention.

Western Individualism: The Basis to Contemporary Occupational Therapy Theory

We may all be observed to *do* and perform activities similarly, but the personal and societal meanings we ascribe and imbue our own activities with are profoundly particular and unique. Where and how do these cultural patterns originate and how are they sustained, despite the pressures to amalgamate or disperse them in this age of information and globalisation? If the stability of cultural patterns were merely explained by physical embodiment as if written into the genetic code of individuals, we would merely need to look no further than the biological explanation. In a social-cultural regard for the explanations for meanings human beings ascribe to what they do, there is a need to reach far into the basic narratives that people hold within themselves that form the keys to understanding existence. People situated in the West may be better at this exercise for their familiarity with the ideas, experiences and sensations of rationalism, monotheism and egalitarianism.

Others may, in their quest to probe social-cultural bases to meanings of *doing*, ponder the matter of cosmological myths or imaginations that people hold for the structure and content of the universe and their imagined places within it. You may have pondered, at one time or another: 'what is the meaning of it all?; why am I here?; where did I come from?; where do we go when we die?; what is the reason for being? is there a God?' In such queries, the views of a larger schema in which meanings are mediated and clarified are being made explicit. These views or narratives are referred to here as 'cosmological myths'[6], and are employed in an attempt to reflect on cultural influences that extend beyond individual physical attribution to include deeper realms of the social.

Readers who have experienced acculturating into very different cultural contexts and have developed not only multi-language fluency and have had intimate involvement in differing religions may attest to the notion that different world views and how we make sense of the world actually do exist. Making sense of or ascribing a certain meaning to phenomena or objects that are experienced or observed is mediated, at least in part, by reflection to some set of reference ideas (construction of normal), sensations (construction of reality) and beliefs (constructions of truth). Independence in self-care might be regarded as a basic necessity within some individualistic social spheres, while it might represent an unfavourable behaviour pattern in a Confucian influenced collectivistic social context. The value of choice or volition of activity might also be interpreted differently according to differing basic social contextual reference points. If different world views indeed exist, there are profound implications for occupational therapy. Practically every concept or idea – from occupation to occupational performance, to client-centred practice, etc., which carry universalistic assumptions yet vary according to culturally situated meanings – is called into reconsideration. While proven to be beneficial in some spheres of experience, the same may result in the alienation and disadvantaging of others abiding in differing views of *normal*, reality and truth.

Occupational therapists in mainstream Western situations have the enviable privilege of anchoring the meaning of occupation and the reason for occupational therapy to essential points of reference in their own spheres of social experience, within their own cosmological myths. The 'occupation' in occupational therapy – resonating as truth for matters of well-being – is explained and anchored to something that is widely regarded and celebrated as the ethos of Western life; 'doing' that is meaningful to a centrally located self.

The East Asian Cosmological Myth

One dominant cosmological myth that is often tied to 'primitive' or ancient societies' interpretations of the cosmos is one that sociologist Robert Bellah[7] referred to as the East Asian Variation of the Cosmological myth. This view of the cosmos and self depicts the universe as a single inseparable entity made up of a constellation of living matter (including human beings, animals, and flora), inanimate matter (rocks, the sky, sea, streams, fallen twigs) and deities arranged more or less in a tightly packed unity (Figure 3.1). You are in the environment as much as the environment is in you. It is important to note that, in this world view, one does not see nor place one's self in the central position of privilege around which the cosmos is supposed to revolve. The self is just another entity that makes up the greater whole, comprised of flora and fauna, other people, deities and inanimate objects.

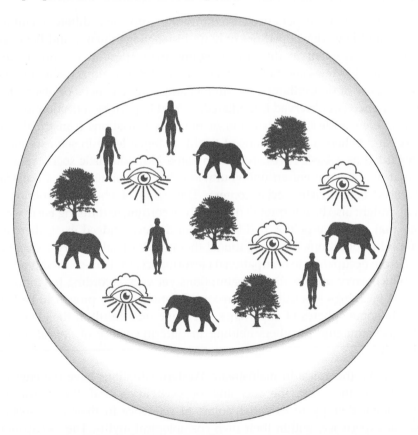

Figure 3.1 Graphic depiction of the East Asian cosmological myth. All elements of the universe are subsumed into one inseparable whole.

An important distinction, according to this construction or understanding of reality and truth, is the inseparable integration of the self with all other elements that make up the whole. Here, Man is not afforded the privilege, nor mandate, to control nature. Issues of control are managed and mediated by the collective. Changes and alteration to any one part of the whole are not contained nor limited in responsibility to one individual but are understood to affect all other aspects of the social frame that they share. The autonomous action of independence is frowned upon and discouraged – it takes on a negative value in this particular world view. One person's unilateral action is a selfish act that threatens to disrupt harmony in the collective system. Thus, an individual who has acculturated into a collectivistic social frame may not demonstrate such a strong drive to initiate changes nor tender any critical thoughts or personal ideas that might potentially upset the harmony idealised in the social frame. In this world view, nature is paramount: constant, encompassing, limiting and enabling, giving and taking away, and humans are just one integrated part of it.

In such views of cosmologies, where all elements of a frame are integrated, the function of occupation as a bridge between self and environment is a non-issue. One is already *there* and no specific effort is prescribed nor required to bridge the two or more parts. 'No less than the trees and the sky, you have a right to be here', goes *the desiderata*[8] which parallels the cosmological views embodied in Eastern philosophical systems. An exploration of Eastern religion and philosophy, such as Mahayana and Zen Buddhism, will reveal a view of the cosmos and the self that is consistent with this variation of the cosmological myth. Occupational therapists working with people representing non-Western cultures may want to investigate these basic narratives more closely. Therapists who have become familiar with the day-to-day life patterns of aboriginal people located around the world can probably attest to the veracity of such ecologically based cosmological myths. One can easily sense that others refer to their relationship with nature in a more integrative way, employing metaphors of nature to explain matters of life and being that differ from the familiar rational narratives Westerners seem to prefer when discussing matters of everyday life. In Western life, self, others and environment are treated as distinct, discretely separate entities, portrayed in relation to each other in industrial metaphors like 'systems' and 'mechanisms' that are rational.

The De-centred Self: Implications for Theories of Human Occupation

There are ramifications of such pervasive cosmological views for the knowledge, theory and practice of our profession. A de-centred self that is embedded in groups and inseparable from nature and environment will consequently have a different constellation of ideas that inform the meanings around 'doing', the meanings of occupation, as well as other essential concepts and ideas in occupational therapy. The idea of client-centred occupational therapy advanced in North America, for example, is plausible in a sphere of social experience and corresponding value patterns in which individual rights of a centrally (imagined and) situated self are accorded primary importance. Not only is the ideology understood and accepted as something that resonates as proper and just and therefore something we ought to incorporate into our ethical practices. Members belonging to the same cultural frame understand how to navigate and enact the behaviours entailed. Here in the West, we are used to speaking about our individual selves, our wants and needs – particularly when asked to do so. And we so easily carry that culturally bound view of *normal* into the lives of people who abide in another socio-cultural sphere of experience, thinking we are doing the right and just thing, and consequently feeling disappointed when those clients seem unable to enact their client-centred roles, perform their independence-driven tasks and play their correct parts.

The value of understanding the client's narrative as precepts to guide occupational therapy intervention, as seen in client-centred approaches to occupational therapy, may be poorly comprehended by people abiding in a social context of collectivism and hierarchy where social stations and power status in a person's life are structured and determined by a vastly different value pattern. The discourse on client-centred occupational therapy, critically examined from a cultural perspective, is only beginning and the issue of cultural relevance will most likely contribute to its further exposition. In the following two chapters, when the explanations of Japanese cultural contexts are expounded on as a rationale for a culturally relevant construction of occupational therapy, other cultural features presented may give a fuller explanation for the futility reported by occupational therapists in other cultural contexts attempting to implement client-centred occupational therapy as constructed in, and defined along, Western spheres of experience.

The Western Variation of the Cosmological Myth

Though the cosmological myth presented represents one particular dominant viewpoint of the 'meaning of it all', the other major variant of it, in its many representations, is perhaps more familiar to people situated in the Western world.

The story of Moses ascending Mount Sinai to meet with Yahweh, as depicted in the Holy scriptures of Judaism and in the Old Testament of the Christian Bible, represents one of the earliest known depictions of a radical reorgani- sation of the 'primitive' (East Asian) cosmological myth. The act of Moses ascending above nature and his people to meet with *the* omnipotent God, on holy ground, high above the wilderness, symbolically illustrates quite clearly a departure from the more 'primitive' world view. The remarkable difference between the East Asian cosmological myth or world view, which configures the universe and all of its elements (including deities, natural flora and fauna, animate and inanimate matter) in one inseparable whole, and the Western variation of it, can be seen in the radical transcendence of an all-powerful God or singular truth over all other elements of the universe. A radical transcendence of a supreme entity parallels a rational separation of the elements of self (like Moses), society (children of Israel), deities (golden calf) and nature (the wilderness) from their former tightly bound unity. Supreme status ascribed to a deity or truth introduces a hierarchical structure – the categorising, naming and organising into graded entities of status along a continuum of power. Whereas nature was a plausible explanation for all phenomena in the former cosmological myth, the Western cosmological myth had exercised boundaries around it (containing all flora and fauna and the environment) and subjugated it to a status below humans.

The transcendence of a single omnipotent deity in Western cosmology[6,9] can also be viewed to correlate symbolically with the individual's transcendence over others (society) and nature (environment) creating an internally (to the self) held view of the self in relation to the world and its concerns (Figure 3.2). In relation to the environment, we derive a sense of individual right and destiny to act on and *occupy* it, having been bestowed dominion over these elements by God. This sense of individual destiny coincides with the unequivocal social assumption of autonomy and independence evident in Western life. We have become familiar with a centrally situated distinct self that supports a developing discourse around how we occupy that distinct self (with meaningful activity) and our environs (through purposeful activity). Disability, itself, is constructed on the discrepancy between personal ability and environmental requirements.

In occupational therapy, independence in daily skills is a universally held and celebrated performance outcome. The requirement to depend on others is pejorative. Dependence is evidence of weakness, of not being competent to control one's circumstances nor fulfill the responsibilities of stewardship of the environment. In Western occupational therapy discourse, these are identified as less desirable states of being that require and deserve amelioration. They set the stage for what constitutes wellness and disability in Western social experience. They also agree well with the principles and structure of contemporary occupational therapy. It seems ironic that our particular placement of emphasis on ability sets the stage or context for its violation.

And What Happened to Nature? Where Did It Go?

The shift from the more 'primitive' and ancient cosmologies of the Eastern world to the rational dissolution of it coincided with another subtle shift in the

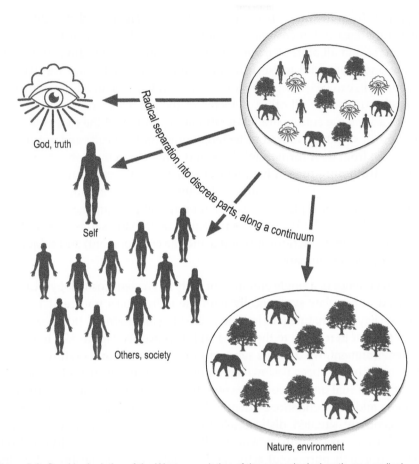

God, truth

Self

Others, society

Nature, environment

Figure 3.2 Graphic depiction of the Western variation of the cosmological myth, as a radical separation of the elements of the universe.

context in which occupational therapists make sense of *doing*. The construction of nature, its structure, content, status and position in relation to human beings and deities, has changed profoundly. Nature has almost disappeared in our Western views of daily life and realities. Of course we talk about it, play in it and routinely watch the weather forecasts but we do so with a particular attitude that differs considerably from those of people in non-industrialised cultures. In a social context of rational consciousness in a post-industrial era bounded by a new myth of purposeful behaviour exemplified in mandates that are typified in terms like efficiency, efficacy, competition and achievement, etc., nature seems to have fallen considerably in status and importance in everyday life. This particular regard for culture is evidenced in its virtual non-existence in contemporary occupational therapy theory and epistemology. Instead of being the basis to all things and phenomena, like the concept of culture, nature has been treated as a somewhat trivial matter. Always there and although a nuisance at times, nature is to be used, altered, managed and exploited to humans' free will. Since the enlightenment, rationalism and the struggle to control nature has continued unabated.

Human beings in industrialised societies continue to devise ways in which to alleviate the resistances that nature presents and to make an easier life despite the environment and circumstances that simply 'happen'. Post-industrial man is only beginning to realise the consequences of neglecting nature and over-exploiting what is a fundamental part of the survival of the human species. Max Weber's essay[10] on 'the Protestant work ethic and the spirit of capitalism' still resonates among concerned scholars today as the industrialised world rips through its natural resources in a consciousness of egocentrism and narcissism, paying little attention to the survival and well-being of generations that are supposed to follow.

I cannot think of any greater threat to the core values of contemporary occupational therapy. Tamper with nature and her resources and consider the consequences to human occupational patterns and the meanings of those occupations. Move the discourse of occupation farther away from nature, towards rationalism and observe the decline of occupation as a potentially meaningful and important entity in the global discourse on health and well-being. The greenhouse effect on climate patterns and changes, global warming melting the polar ice fields and changing the delicate ecological balance that keep our seasons in place, modifying food and organisms genetically, stand to alter profoundly what we eat and the way we eat, and the efficient means by which the world's forests and fish stocks are depleted. Affluent nations continue on their relentless narcissistic occupations of consumption and exploitation, all to the potential peril of the nature that sustains the very existence of *Homo sapiens* and other life forms.

Instead of being regarded as the basis and explanation of all phenomena and things, nature has been relegated to a lower status – to be controlled, managed and tended for the purpose of production (and profit). There has been an important subtle shift from a relationship of harmony and balance between nature and humans to one in which man has been appointed to a higher rung of privilege and situated at the centre of the universe. Following industrialisation, and now on into the age of information, 'primitive' grand narratives for life have 'evolved' to supposed advanced metaphors of machines and mechanical systems. It is certainly sexier, with the times, and more credible to base your profession's guiding narratives on images (metaphors) of science, medicine and technology over something as ubiquitous, ancient and basic as 'nature'. Yet, the ascendance of man and subjugation of nature[11] is arbitrary and but an illusion. The cycle of birth and death, like the unremitted cycles of days and nights, tides and seasons, the fallow of winter and the rejuvenation of spring, or the ferocity of hurricanes, tsunamis and earthquakes, have yet to be controlled. What goes up still comes down, and rivers continue their long journeys from mountain glaciers and tarns towards the distant sea. Nature still is an important and powerful determinant of people's well-being, despite mankind's illusory assertions of dominion over it.

As occupational therapy scholarship continues along the path towards greater legitimacy and credibility, its membership should at least be cognisant of the tensions that draw it in one direction rather than another. Legitimacy in the world of medical scientific research is what our academics seek. Clinicians and practitioners in the meantime, while pursuing best practice and striving to be better consumers of medical scientific knowledge, should ponder the hidden values of life and shared experiences and meanings of our clientele. It would be tragic to lose credibility with occupational therapy clients and communities. To gain legitimacy in the world of science yet lose that legitimacy among those we endeavour to serve will ensure that occupational therapy will not advance to be the beneficial movement that it was meant to be.

The emergence of the Western cosmological myth has advanced a narrative that has subordinated nature from its former central location of concern to the place under the foot of *Homo sapiens*. Whether or not cosmological myths and particular world views have any bearing on a given social group's value and belief systems, certain traits or conceptualisations have been raised often in the literature to describe Western individualism in light of its contexts of rational world views. Some of these concepts describe the modal Western individual as being *analytic*[12,13,14], *monotheistic*[15,6,16], *materialistic*[12] and *rationalistic*[17].

Concepts that describe a particular attitude towards doing, such as *unilateral determinism*[18], *self-efficacy*[19], and *personal causation*[20] reflect a construal of individualistic intention and construction of 'self' in relation to environment. In Western spheres of experience, the occupation of one's environs through purposeful action is often viewed as a right and imperative. It assumes, as Lebra[18] had postulated, that the prime mover for one's actions lies within the individual for the Westerner, with the ultimate objective being to gain competence and independence by establishing control over one's circumstances (Figure 3.3). In this attitude towards human agency, responsibility for

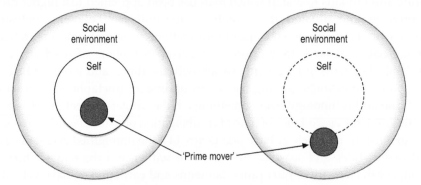

Figure 3.3 Location of the 'prime mover' in relation to self and social environment. In individual-centred societies (left), the prime mover is located within the self, while in collective-oriented societies (right), the prime mover is located towards the periphery of the self into the domain of the collective.

success and failure tend to fall on the individual more than the surrounding social context.

Western individualism on a micro level is congruent with *monotheism* – the tendency to support a 'closed system cosmology' where limits are, on a macro level, convergent to a single truth or omnipotent deity[6]. The congruence between a closed system theology and a closed system personology – where phenomena are viewed to be accountable to a single set of laws or moral standards, is evident in virtually all modes and explanations of Western life[21]. Modern science, with all of its positivistic and empirical principles thought to originate from such a world view, reifies a universe that is rationally constructed. The universe is configured in a logical sequence and therefore reducible to a single basic truth. The orderly division and categorisation of reality is not only pertinent to physical 'real' things, but presumed also to constitute the structure of immaterial things such as thoughts, ideas and memories[12]. Thus the Western individual is construed to be especially analytical, preferring a view of reality as an aggregation of parts (that fit together in some ultimately logical pattern). Western theorists and researchers have thus sought to 'objectify' the world in a particular way, seeking to reduce the complexities of human thought and action into more linear, logical explanations.

The tendency to construct the world in an analytical, particulate manner, which is congruent with a particulate[22] view of self, society and nature, represents an important tenet of occupational therapy philosophy. That problematic tenet is the objectification of 'external' objects as existing separately from the observer (Figure 3.4). The view of the environment (both social and physical, etc.) seen in opposition to the self (connected through 'occupation') rather than viewing the environment[23,22] as just one part of the same unified whole, holds profound implications for whether people of other cultures[24] can share and abide by Western occupational therapists' interpretations of occupation and its supposed essentiality to well-being.

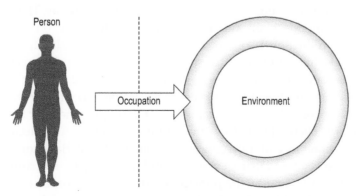

Figure 3.4 Occupation constructed as the link between the discretely defined and separated person and environment, in Western narratives of agency and self-determinism.

Thus, Westerners and their ideas about human agency are, from time to time, considered to be (overly) rational. In this epistemological leaning, all phenomena, including human agency and praxis, can be reflectively and systematically investigated and explained by some rational logic. Human performance qualifies as occupation when we interpret it as meaningful; when the means of a task can be tied to some reasonable end. The importance of tying one's action or 'doing', rationally, to some future objective, orients one temporally towards the future.

On which world views are current rehabilitation and occupational therapy models based? And what are the implications when these models are applied outside of their original cultural contexts? Postulates regarding the congruence between Western world views and occupational therapy theory should be readily evident in occupational therapy theory, particularly those conceptual models that purport to explain human agency and its qualities. The Model of Human Occupation[25] (MOHO), and the Canadian Model of Occupational Performance[26] (CMOP) are briefly examined here to illuminate how culture is implicit in the structure and contents of these theoretical cognitions. It should be noted that the earliest, substantive descriptions of these conceptual models are being purposely referred to for the purpose of situating the genesis of these ideas into a historical and cultural context. That these models undergo adaptations better to meet the changing requirements of their respective dynamically changing social contexts is testament to the thesis of this chapter; that meaning and its explanations are culturally situated.

Until recently, the issue of culture, which has been regarded as a secondary consideration or afterthought, was never seriously considered to be embedded within theory itself. These are but two of many conceptual models used by occupational therapists, and the analyses from a cultural perspective that ensue are unfairly brief. However, this is merely a start and an initial foray into understanding the cultural dimensions of occupational therapy conceptual frameworks. These models have proven their relevance and effectiveness in many contexts of occupational therapy practice and have contributed significantly towards occupational therapy's development to this day. The argument put forward in this book and in an emerging discourse on culture and knowledge production is one of cultural relevance and situated meaning. These models, like all models that seek to conceptualise social processes and phenomena, emerge from a particular world view and context of shared meanings. They are limited, like most social frameworks in generalisability and research efforts should also examine their appropriateness for local clients as well as for clients located in other cultural contexts. As reflected in the following section, a cultural analysis of theoretical material should look at validity – especially construct validity and whether the structure of and explanations postulated by the principles formed by the constructs are valid. Many of the instruments that develop from conceptual models carry within their contents and protocols a basic set of assumptions born from their parent models. Whenever therapists use these materials and come away perplexed for why things did not go as well as expected, a common tendency is locate the problem in the client rather than a fundamental flaw or problem of cultural relevance in the instrument and the *theory* it is based on.

A review of the model of human occupation[20] reveals that General Systems Theory[27,28] (GST) was chosen as the framework on which the concepts of this model were to be structured. The model depicts humans as open systems involved in an intercourse with the surrounding physical and social environment. The basic tenet to this interpretation of human action was that humans had an innate drive to master (control) their environments. Their subsequent actions in the world were modified by an internal executive order of cognition, which ultimately assembled, modified and enacted performance. *Volition, Habituation* and *Performance* comprised the three main occupational performance components residing in the *open system*[25]. Subsumed in the concept of volition are sub-concepts perceived to be resident in the individual such as, 'personal causation', 'values' and 'interests'. Under the sub-concept of 'personal causation', the concepts of 'self-efficacy' and one's 'knowledge of capacity' (to perform) are contained. Acting upon the environment would result in feedback and other cues from the environment, which would input into the system, pass through the executive functions and output again into the environment, forming a loop. *Functional* states of the individual would be characterised by smooth cycling and equilibrium in the human–environment continuum, while uneven, blocked cycling and imbalance would characterise *occupational dysfunctional* states. The occupational therapist, in using this model, would endeavour to assist the patient to gain a better equilibrium with his or her environments by maximising performance in any part of the human–environment continuum.

The model of human occupation's structure and concepts, and metaphoric representation of human agency depicted in a mechanical systems arrangement, reflects virtually all of the descriptors of the modal Western tendencies and cosmologies presented above. The 'self' is depicted as solitary and placed in the centre of the 'system'. The transcendence of self over an environment that is distinctly set in opposition is also evident. Successful human agency is conceptualised as a state of efficacy in which a person can exercise one's determination to act on the environment and control one's circumstances. 'Control' in this interpretation is set synonymously with 'balance'. The compartmentalisation of the various concepts and sub-concepts systematically working together in logical order is reminiscent of depictions of Western individuals as *analytic, materialistic* and *rationalistic*.

The Canadian Model of Occupational Performance[29,1] is yet another prominent model to emerge in the latter half of the 20th century. Like the Model of Human Occupation, this conceptual model has undergone some changes and development of both internal concepts and structural principles between the constructs. The adaptations and amendments to any model or depiction of phenomena so that the model remains potent to explain phenomena in a way that remains meaningful to the population that it is meant for, is testament to the cultural relationship between models and their creators and users. Spheres of experience vary and societal changes occur to demonstrate the dynamic and changing character of culture along the lines of time and place. As with all models, the professional should exercise a critical eye when regarding and using these theoretical materials. The astute, culturally aware therapist may ponder: 'why were these constructs and concepts chosen or decided upon?' 'why are the constructs tied together in this way?' and 'do the constructs mean what they were meant to mean when the model is applied to its intended target clientele?'

Three concentric circles representing components of the human-occupation-environment system graphically depict the Canadian model, which borrows some of its features from Reed and Sanderson's[30] previous work on occupational performance. The 'individual' is represented by the innermost circle and is conceptualised to consist of four parts: spiritual, physical, mental and socio-cultural. Onlookers may want to ponder critically why the centrally situated individual is constructed in this particular quadrate. What was the basis to this particular representation of the human system, and does this tell us anything about the cultural perspectives of the model's creators?

As with each of the concepts used to describe the individual, the cultural construction of concepts is evident. The concept of spirituality arguably represents the basic problem confronting issues of meaning. If the arguments put forward in the pages of this book are at all plausible, then one can easily see that varying spheres of experience of people around spirituality will render the concept problematic whenever universal meaning is sought. Who makes the decision regarding what the definition of a concept should be? If conceptual models are to be relevant and powerful tools for enabling clients of occupational therapy, it should be appropriate for occupational therapy theorists to develop concepts and their meanings with primary input and direction from their client populations.

The outermost circle represents the environment and is conceptualised into four parts: physical, social, cultural and institutional. Between the innermost circle (the individual) and the outermost circle (the environment) lies the middle concentric circle, which has been conceptualised, as 'areas of occupational performance'. These areas of performance are divided into three parts: self-care, productivity and leisure. Occupational performance is depicted in this model as the balance between individual and environment. The interaction between self and environs is through action (occupation). A deficit in one's ability to act according to will results in dysfunction and an upset of systematic balance.

Occupational therapists work to identify the points contributing to imbalance in the system and use activity therapeutically to strengthen and re-balance the system. Thus intervention strategies are geared towards restoring one's mastery over the environment by adjusting individual or environmental attributes. Once again, the primacy of the individual as agent of change in relation to the environment is strongly represented. The concepts and conceptualisation of both the individual and environment into limited, discrete components is evident and affords us a view into how the authors constructed the concept of occupational performance along the concepts of individual agency, environment and the utility and meaning of action.

What is evident in these constructions of well-being is the notion that personal achievement or self-actualisation represent the acme of human strivings and that these ideals are derived through a process of exploration and competence. 'Mastery' of self and the environment (nature) become equated with healthy states of being. These occupational therapy conceptual models represent and reify Western ideals of health defined along independent, individualistic and rationalistic proclivities. How appropriate, then, are these depictions of health for societies that abide by very different social and cultural constructions of reality?

Students of occupational therapy are encouraged to look at the culture embedded in contemporary occupational therapy models and to determine how closely the structure and content of the models resonate with the cultures of the therapist and client. Applying concepts and principles without such due consideration can render occupational therapy with potentially disastrous effects. Culturally misguided procedures can result in disadvantaging the client by disrespecting the client's world of meanings.

Philosophical Positions

The juxtaposed presentation of two example world views presented in this chapter were offered to challenge the explanatory power of universal narratives and to point towards the need for culturally specific conceptualisations of occupation, theory and models.

The East Asian version of the cosmological myth, discussed earlier, suggests that modal Asian and Western people may perceive the world quite differently. Instead of perceiving the world as rationally separated, many East Asians may take the perspective that places nature, self and society in a 'closed' tightly integrated whole. There are no social-structural after-effects of a radical transcendence of a single God, single truth or single moral code. Rather than linear ties of loyalty and trust extending (vertically) towards a single deity or universal ideal, they settle into a complex, flexible constellation of (horizontal) relations. With regard to human behaviour, the social

49

(in absence of an omnipotent deity) becomes the entity by which all things are valuated and judged. Persistence of the cosmological myth in Eastern concept-ualisations of nature, self and society, compared to the Western transcendent, separated version of it, can be correlated to certain observable social-structural patterns.

This world view, for example, may limit the conceptualisation of the central-ity of 'self' in the universe as well as deflect reliance and attribution of accomplishment away from a solitary, centrally situated 'me'. The reflective 'Westerner' may have difficulty regarding this sensation of being as remark-able – as thinking, acting, and relating to all things in nature and the universe, from a central reference point of 'me' – is and has always been normal. And instead of a monotheistic view of an ultimate singular truth, the Eastern cosmological view places deities together with humans and nature in a tightly bound singular entity, creating a polytheism in which multiple truths can coincide. In the Western sense of the cosmos, the transcendent individual is afforded an elevated vantage point from which to view and judge all matter according to a single, internally reflected, universally applicable moral code. For the polytheistic Easterner, no such perch exists from which to ultimately judge matters. Judgement and interpretation of truth and right is situational, reflected to referent elements in the vicinity of the phenomena rather than to a universal interpretation of truth and moral right that transcends local context. In such relational contexts, the notion of grand theories or all encompassing explanations of phenomena are unimaginable and practically untenable.

Similar versions of such a naturalistic world view form the basis to collectivist social structures described in many Asian, African and Aboriginal societies. They represent particular contexts of meaning that become awkward substrates for setting individualistic, independence-oriented constructions of occupation. Occupation, as with so many of occupational therapy's contem-porary core concepts and prominent narratives are currently bound by a certain world view and corresponding value pattern. In this way, the profes-sion is challenged to make its ideas, ideology, theory and the practices that follow, relevant to many, many groups of people. By treating culture as an individually bound feature of the client as opposed to a fundamental element of occupational therapy itself, it has fallen far short of any ideas that would make it truly inclusive, ethical and just for its clientele. These issues raise questions about the client-centred practice of occupational therapy to another level of consideration. What was previously regarded to be a dynamic located at the nexus of therapist and client, client-centred practice issues are now expanded to include the interface of occupational therapy's embedded culture and the world of the client's culture.

In Japanese social contexts, for example, the 'de-centralised' conceptualisation of self is seen to permit a 'situation ethic'[31,32] to determine behaviour whereby the social situation (referred to as 'frame' or 'ba' by Nakane[33]) and not the centrally constructed self, strongly influences the interpretation, initiation and shape of human agency. With emphasis placed on horizontal social relations tied to 'frame', a social or group-focused norm gains prominence over an individual-focused norm where matters pertaining to existentialism and identity are contingent on 'doing'. Thus, Lebra's[18] suggestion that the 'prime mover', which is located internally in most Westerners, is seen to be located external to the self, in the social 'frame', for the modal Japanese person.

So much of the discourse on human occupation is individualistic and therefore reflexive. The notion of deriving meaning from what we do is tacit for most people who abide in a monistic, egocentric view of the world. Many non-Western occupational therapists and their clients have trouble participating in such a perspective of self and the meaning of action owing to the lack of such experiences and interpretation of phenomena in their own realities and experiences of the social. For many non-mainstream Western people, the meanings attributed to personal agency and phenomena are situational, allocentrically influenced and vary from circumstance to circumstance. Truth and the meaning of doing may be greatly influenced by the social surroundings and the situation of the agent vis-à-vis the environment.

In the Japanese collective experience, more than the self, the group in which one holds membership is agent. When the social frame takes precedence over individual attribute, the realisation of personal goals and social roles are constructed to come about by a different dynamic. Achievement is rarely a solitary attribute but a result of self, the collective and nature. In the West, there is the notion that we can affect the state of nature (and health) through our actions *as energised by mind and will*[34]. Hence, the belief that we can *achieve* societal roles and attain success by striving intelligently and unilaterally persists. The progression of *doing, being and becoming,* as Wilcock iterated, need not be questioned. In Japanese social experience, being and becoming are not necessarily contingent on one's effort or skill. Nature, which includes the collective, encompasses the self as a unified whole, ultimately explains success and failure and practically every outcome. In the East, the concepts of fate or karma often provide powerful explanation for all phenomenal outcomes. These differences between individualist and collectivist views towards occupational performance outcomes can be practically seen in cross-cultural interactions, such as international sporting events like the Olympics. Westerners may find it intriguing to compare the content of interviews given by high performance athletes to television media reporters following a successful outcome. Japanese athletes will, almost certainly, begin their interview with expressions of sincere gratitude to the fans, team mates, support staff, coaches and, practically everyone else, for the successes achieved. This is not only because of social convention in a collectivist society but also because the athlete himself or herself basically believes that the success achieved was the result of many factors that coincided at that time and place. And in normal circumstances, the sensation of self as central and transcendent over all other concern as it seems to be in Western spheres of experiences is not as strongly felt in a Japanese social context. Victory was not necessarily achieved because the solitary self was able to produce a supreme personal effort or that God had willed it to be. In contrast, the Western victor's assertive, enthusiastic rationalisations attributing victory to a supreme personal effort or to God, with numerous reflective 'I' statements, appear immature and overly egocentric when judged from a collectivist-bound value pattern.

Belonging, Being and Doing

In a collective valued society where one is accountable to one's social relationships over and above some single truth or universally held moral standard, *belonging* rather than *doing* becomes the social ethos. Matters of identity and meaning are ascribed in collective rather than in introspective processes. To be cast out of one's group can result in the devastating experience of having one's identity and reason for existing invalidated. In these societies, given the value pattern around social processes and what is worth doing, the collective is considered more agent than the individual. Hence the drive to be independent and autonomous, so dominant in modern rehabilitation and occupational therapy, might appear strange or novel judged from a social backdrop that values social dependence and interdependence. In this context of collective belonging, the progression of *becoming, being and doing* is a more convincing model to explain the dynamic between doing and being. Roles are bestowed by the group and received by the individual, for no individual is considered greater than the collective. And once the role is made explicit, the self emerges to carry out the mandate of the collective. This is fulfillment in Japanese social life and the acme of modal Japanese agency. Japan's rise from the ashes of the Second World War to its place as one of the world's strongest economies can be attributed, at least partly, to the efficacy of industrial companies fuelled by this social value pattern around collective agency.

More examples and discussion of the Japanese social will follow in the next chapter to elucidate further the idea of relation between theory and cultural context.

Towards Context Based Conceptualisations of Occupation

Often the culture embedded in our own views of reality goes unnoticed. The features of our shared experiences remain unremarkable to all who belong to the same frame because the perch, from which we universally judge other elements of the world around us, itself, is exempted from scrutiny. Many simply never notice this platform of privilege from which we construct the world around us. If we can, for a moment, lower that perch and descend our point of reference to view and appreciate *other* world views and perspectives of reality, we gain insight into our own culture and our own particular ways of seeing and knowing.

Currently, the critical examination of culture subsumed in our profession's fundamental thoughts and language remain underdeveloped and particularly biased towards shared meanings and interpretations of phenomena germane to Western spheres of experience. In this chapter, some of the more prominent descriptions of Western social proclivities were raised into view. The descriptions included individualistic, autonomous, analytic, monotheistic, materialistic and rationalistic leanings germane to Western cultural lenses. These limited concepts were also explained in relation to possible differences in world views that have a bearing on how one constructs the individual in relation to the social and to elements of the environment. How this fundamental view of reality is configured can have a profound effect on if and how people ascribe meaning to their actions and place in the world. In other words, these basic world views have a fundamental bearing on the meaning of occupation. A cosmological view that constructs self as equal in status to and inseparably 'one' with the environment challenges the claim that we occupy our environs through occupation. Self-deterministic notions of unilaterally controlling life circumstances through occupation are lost on people who ascribe to more naturalistic viewpoints of reality and who are oriented towards a harmonious existence with nature and its circumstances.

How might the problem of theory and knowledge systems out of sync with the complex cultural contexts of the client's daily life be evidenced? In collective, Confucian hierarchically oriented societies like those of Asia, for example, a well-meaning therapist working with an elderly man in an extended care facility may unwittingly negate a lifetime of meaningful experiences and skills for *being* by guiding him through a care mandate founded on and informed by North American value patterns and views of reality. Armed with theory and instruments based on Western narratives that reflect middle-class values and realities, the therapist may be coercing the client into social requirements that are poorly understood and run counter to context for *being*. The yearning to belong, to depend, to be in harmony with his circumstances and carry out the role that he has been given in his station in time (just like they may have been for centuries) are being intruded upon, frustrated and dismantled by an ideology based on the predication of individualism and independence/autonomy, made explicit in concepts like *personal causation, occupational performance*, and the battery of proprietary assessments that follows.

Problems of cultural incongruence are often overlooked for the sake of communities wanting the latest and 'best' advancements from the West. And when these ideas and materials are exported under the pretences that they are beneficial, emancipating, empowering and restoring, it is difficult to place a critical barrier in the way. Those who are fearful of being left behind the global economy and state of technology may actually put out the welcome mat and not necessarily see it as an *intrusion*. Some may indeed benefit but the parallels to colonialism from past times are once again recalled. There is always the danger of bringing in our culture and therefore our standards of behaviour and meanings that can disrupt people's normal ways of life. In the local cultural context, we may actually be modelling and nurturing behaviours that will disadvantage people in their societies. In this way, occupational therapy can potentially oppress rather than empower, encumber rather than emancipate, and disable rather than restore.

If meaning in occupation is deemed important to members of this profession, then the issue of culture should be of primary concern. When we take occupational therapy into the lives of people living outside of our own familiar social contexts, we need to allow the insiders of client groups to understand and dictate the terms by which occupational therapy is assembled and delivered. Occupational therapists are implored to go beyond the requirements of conventional cultural competence and recognise the cultural construction of occupational therapy itself, and all of its subsumed philosophies, theories and epistemologies. Failure to do so will ensure that occupational therapy will fall far short of its mandate to enable people through meaningful action.

REFERENCES

1 Canadian Association of Occupational Therapists. Enabling Occupation: An Occupational Therapy Perspective. Toronto: CAOT Publications; 1997

2 Christiansen C. Defining lives; occupation as identity: an essay on competence, coherence, and the creation of meaning. 1999 Eleanor Clarke Slagle Lectureship. American Journal of Occupational Therapy 1999; 53(6):547–558

3 Mead G. Mind, Self, and Society. Chicago: University of Chicago Press; 1967

4 Piaget J. The Construction of Reality in the Child. New York: Ballantine; 1954

5 Wilcock A. Reflections on doing, being, and becoming. Canadian Journal of Occupational Therapy 1998; 65:248–256

6 Bellah R. Beyond Belief: Essays on Religion in a Post Traditional World. New York: Harper & Row; 1991

7 Bellah RN. Tokugawa Religion. Glencoe: The Free Press; 1957

8 Ehrmann M. Desiderata. Los Angeles: Brooke House; 1972

9 Berque A. Identification of the self in relation to the environment. In: Rosenberger N (ed). Japanese Sense of Self. Cambridge: Cambridge University Press; 1992; 93–104

[10] Weber M. The Protestant Ethic and the Spirit of Capitalism. London: Allen and Unwin; 1904–5 (1976)

[11] Scott CH. Knowledge construction among Cree hunters: metaphors and literal understanding. Journal de la Société des Américanistes 1989; 75:193–208

[12] Johnson F. Dependency and Japanese Socialization: Psychoanalytic and Anthropological Investigations into Amae. New York: New York University Press; 1993

[13] Porkert M. The Theoretical Foundation of Chinese Medicine. Boston: Massachusetts Institute of Technology Press; 1974

[14] Gregory-Smith D. Science and technology in East Asia. Philosophy East and West 1979; 29:221–236

[15] DeVos G. Dimensions of self in Japanese culture. In: Marsella A, DeVos G, Hsu F (eds), Culture and Self: Asian and Western Perspectives. New York: Tavistock; 1985; 32–88

[16] Miller D. The New Polytheism. New York: Harper & Row; 1974

[17] Gans H. Middle American Individualism. New York: The Free Press; 1988

[18] Lebra S. Japanese Patterns of Behavior. Honolulu: University of Hawaii Press; 1976

[19] Bandura A. Self-efficacy: toward a unifying theory of behavioral change. Psychological Review 1977; 84:191–215

[20] Kielhofner G. A Model of Human Occupation: Theory and Application. Baltimore: Williams and Wilkins; 1985

[21] Bellah RN, Madsen R, Sullivan WM, Swidler A, Tipton SM. Habits of the Heart: Individualism and Commitment in American Life. Berkeley, CA: University of California Press; 1985

[22] Ellen RF. The cognitive geometry of nature: a contextual approach. In: Descola P, Pálsson G (eds), Nature and Society: Anthropological Perspectives. London: Routledge; 1996; 103–123

[23] Ingold T. The Perception of the Environment: Essays on Livelihood, Dwelling and Skill. London: Routledge; 2000

[24] Hallowell AI. Ojibwa ontology, behavior, and world view. In: Diamond S (ed.), Culture in History: Essays in Honor of Paul Radin. New York: Columbia University Press; 1960; 19–52

[25] Kielhofner G, Burke JP. A model of human occupation. Part 1: Conceptual framework and content. American Journal of Occupational Therapy 1980; 34:572–581

[26] Department of National Health and Welfare & Canadian Association of Occupational Therapists. Guidelines for the Client-Centred Practice of Occupational Therapy, Cat.H39–33/1983. Ottawa: Department of National Health and Welfare; 1983

[27] von Bertalanffy L. An outline of general systems theory. British Journal for the Philosophy of Science 1950; 1:134–164

[28] Parsons T. The Structure of Social Action. New York: McGraw-Hill; 1937

[29] Canadian Association of Occupational Therapists. Occupational Therapy Guide-lines for Client Centred Practice. Toronto: CAOT Publications; 1986

[30] Reed K, Sanderson S. Concepts of Occupational Therapy. Baltimore: Williams and Wilkins; 1980

[31] DeVos G. The relation of guilt toward parents to achievement and arranged marriage among the Japanese. Psychiatry 1960; 23:287–301

[32] Lebra ST. Self in Japanese culture. In: Rosenberger NR (ed.), Japanese Sense of Self. New York: Cambridge University Press; 1992

[33] Nakane C. Tate shakai no ningen kankei [Human Relations in a Vertical Society]. Tokyo: Kodansha; 1970

[34] Reilly M. Occupational therapy can be one of the great ideas of 20th century medicine. American Journal of Occupational Therapy 1962; 16:1–9

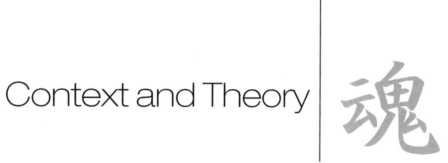

Context and Theory

Cultural Antecedents of the Kawa Model Part 1

魂

In the previous chapters, the issue of culture as a fundamental basis to a profession's knowledge base (what occupational therapists consider to be worth knowing), theory (how occupational therapists explain what they do) and practice (what occupational therapists actually do) was presented. Before a discussion of the need for culturally relevant models can proceed, there is a need to explore the relation between particular cultural contexts and the theoretical materials that are meant to guide practice. So much of the culture within our own contexts of experience is difficult to make explicit as it remains hidden in the familiar and normal. The brief analyses of MOHO and CMOP in the previous chapter might have struck some occupational therapists as being rather crude and extreme in many spots. However, those particular observations were drawn from, and perhaps made possible by, a different contextual vantage or cultural lens. The tacit agreement on independence and autonomy of Western life and rehabilitation ideals often appear to be remarkably egocentric from a collectivistic value orientation where interdependence is a commonly celebrated ideal. So the normal and mundane in one cultural setting can appear to be abnormal and remarkable in another cultural setting.

In these middle chapters, the perches upon which we stand to view and make sense of the other are turned around. We proceed from a critical evaluation of contemporary conceptual models and the contexts in which they have developed, to an examination or description of an Eastern social context to gain a better sense of what kind of conceptual models and theory might safely fit such cultural contexts. In the process, occupational therapists may gain further appreciation for why a group of Japanese clinicians could conclude that contemporary models learned rote thus far were problematic to their practice and profession. These points of critical reflection will hopefully stimulate some thoughts – whether you are situated in Asia or not – about what occupational therapists may have to do in developing their theory in the coming era, to ensure that their profession and practice are meaningful, useful, equitable, enabling and truly empowering.

In this discussion of culture and its purported relation to knowledge and theory, a thesis running through all of it is the assertion that conceptual models cannot serve as definitive, universal narratives on occupation unless occupation is delimited to specific Western spheres of experience. The Kawa model, in its original form, must be understood in regard to its original contexts of genesis. By understanding the relationship between models and their contextual origins, the occupational therapist can make decisions regarding whether to use the model in its original form, change it to suit the needs of the client's contexts of meanings or put it aside for a more appropriate framework.

While encountering these explanations of the Japanese social, readers may find themselves juxtaposing their own experiences of the social in their various cultural settings to those of the Japanese. It may be helpful to keep pondering whether the occupational therapy knowledge and theory learned until now could be applied in differing cultural settings. Readers may ask what happens to the meanings and applications of constructs when they cross cultural borders. What are the prevailing narratives of Japanese people, and how do these differ from your own and from contemporary occupational therapy's? And lastly, you may have some ideas about what culturally relevant and culturally safe conceptual models for this particular clientele might look like.

For this discussion, descriptions by Japanese social scientists and commentators about the Japanese social are depicted in explanations and apologies for certain modal behaviour patterns and social structure. By far, this should not to be considered a definitive explanation of the Japanese social, for even this analysis is conducted through fixed cultural lenses bounded by place and time. They are offered, nonetheless, as points of comparison and contrast with the various social and cultural settings the reader may be familiar with. The ultimate exercise here is to imagine what forms and meanings of occupational therapy might best suit the contexts for well-being and health in a particular cultural context. And though the structure of the cultural analyses presented here is drawn along the boundaries of ethnicity and race, the reader is directed to use the broader definition of culture offered – that culture is more about shared spheres of experiences and meanings, when making the comparative juxtapositions and pondering the meanings and structure of culturally relevant occupation.

Japan: Occupations in the Land of the Rising Sun

Japan's 120 million people form a part of Asia's collective population estimated to be over 3.3 billion people[1] – almost half of the world's population. Asia's varied cultures represent a pertinent testing ground for occupational therapy's universality because, as a whole, it has evolved its own distinct philosophies, value patterns, moral and ethical systems and epistemologies, separate from the Western world[2]. Just as Asian nations have had to reconcile the sharp intrusions of modernisation and Western cultural forms, over the past century, Japan has had to deal with the systematic transplantation of occupational therapy with all of its subsumed philosophies, values, moral and ethical systems and epistemology from the West over the past 40 years. Japan's is arguably one of the fastest proliferating occupational therapy concerns in the world, with occupational therapy education programmes expanding at a near exponential rate in the past decade. During the preparation of this book, there were 140 schools of occupational therapy meeting the requirements for accreditation according to the guidelines put forward by the World Federation of Occupational Therapists (WFOT).

In relation to the world views and construction of self referred to in the previous chapters, modal Japanese interpretations of being in the world are more consistent with what Bellah[3] referred to as the East Asian variation of the cosmological myth. Such a world view typically places nature, self and society in a 'closed' tightly integrated whole. That is, nature, deities, self and society would be viewed and experienced as an inseparable unified whole. There are no social-structural after-effects of a radical transcendence of a single God, single truth or single moral code. Rather than linear ties of loyalty and trust extending (vertically) towards a single deity or universal ideal, they settle into a complex, flexible constellation of (horizontal) relations. With regard to human behaviour, the *social* (in absence of an omnipotent deity) becomes the entities by which all things are valuated and judged. Persistence of this cosmological myth in Eastern conceptualisations of nature, self and society, compared to the Western transcendent, separated version of it, can be correlated to certain observable social-structural patterns in Japanese social frames. This world view, for example, may limit the conceptualisation of the centrality of 'self' in the universe as well as deflecting reliance and attribution of accomplishment away from a solitary, centrally situated self.

Macro-Sociological Perspectives on Japanese Patterns of Behaviour and Meaning

Many Japanese people, who hold such a collectivistic world view, will most likely agree with the observation that they are not comfortable making 'I' statements frequently or talking at length about one's self. The self is almost always seen in relation to or in the context of other members of his or her identified group. This feature of Japanese shared experience is frequently ignored by some observers who attempt to make sense of Japanese behaviour patterns using individual-centred, commonly shared Western spheres of experience and associated meanings.

Part of a Japanese business man's preoccupation with reading a business card with the respectful gesture of holding the card with both of his hands is to make sure that he is fully cognisant and appreciative of the other's identity and place – in the context of the organisation to which they belong. Due care is taken to confirm the rank and department to which the other belongs, and never is the face of the card written on in the presence of its owner, nor is the card immediately filed away. Doing so would be interpreted as a gesture of deliberate disrespect. A large measure of the respect, power and status an individual holds is directly determined by the social context or organisation to which he belongs. No matter how individually talented or incompetent he or she happens to be, these individual attributes are lesser points of concern than the group in which he holds membership. The same conditions are socialised into practically every facet of Japanese social life. The same value pattern and behaviours around identity can be observed among school children, housewife gatherings, recreational clubs and even occupational therapists.

Such a 'de-centralised' conceptualisation of self purportedly permits a 'situation ethic'[4] to determine behaviour whereby the social situation (referred to as 'frame' or 'ba' by Nakane[5]), and not a centrally constructed *self*, strongly influences the interpretation, initiation and shape of human agency. And with emphasis placed on horizontal social relations tied to 'frame', a social-focused norm gains prominence over an individual-focused norm where matters pertaining to existentialism and identity are contingent on 'doing'. Thus Lebra's[4] suggestion that the 'prime mover', which is located internally in most Westerners, is seen to be located external to the self in the social 'frame', for the modal Japanese person.

Takie Sugiyama Lebra[4] had also recognised the significance of cosmology in shaping values and social behaviour. In particular, she draws on Japanese myth and cosmology as part of a framework of influences that precede the peculiar Japanese form of situational ethic and structure of morality. Two well-known mythological tales from antiquity, the *Kojiki* and *Nihongi* are quoted from Pelzel's[6] work in which it is noted that the mythmakers appear to have an earth-bound imagination. Supernatural beings are often brought down to human status, sharing the earth dwelling and *this-worldly* way of life with their human counterparts (p. 9).

Other Japanese scholars have commented on the consequences of the East Asian cosmology in Japanese experiences and interpretations of reality. Haga[7], a well-known Japanese scholar purported to be influential in Japanese pre-war education, commented that the Japanese remained 'this-worldly' even after the importation of Buddhism, which introduced another world of prior and future existences. The Japanese seem to have retained a 'here-and-now' temporal orientation to insure their 'this-worldly' welfare but they have apparently never been sympathetic to the Buddhist alienation from this life. Haga points out that Japanese often show a fickle attitude towards Buddhism, witnessed in casual sacrilegious comments about 'hotoke' (Buddhas) in proverbs, folk sayings and comedies.

Similarly for the Japanese, as Lebra[4] points out, humans have no claim to superiority over other animals; even inanimate things behave like humans. Pelzel[6] adds that: 'Imbued with a sense of harmony between the supernatural and the natural, and between man and other forms of life, the ancient Japanese seem to have been indifferent to ontological speculation of the universe and human existence' (p. 86). Japanese culture has since been exposed to foreign cultures, such as Chinese, Buddhist, European and the West, but they have not changed fundamentally in this respect.

East Asian Cosmology and Japanese Morality

This cosmological humanism expressed in Japan may not be said to accord with social relativism in that social relativism demands that all elements of the universe be related horizontally and mutually, and that they share the same human status rather than being hierarchically controlled with the ultimate keeper of the order (God) at the top of morality. The Western tenets of democracy, whereby all men are believed to be created equal before God and therefore accountable to a single moral code, is lost on many Japanese people. The clear-cut dualisms of Western 'unilateral determinism', such as 'good/bad', 'right/wrong', etc., that is characteristic of unilateral determinism, is not congenial to the Japanese sense of morality. For Japanese people, Lebra[4] reiterates, goodness or badness are relative matters. They are relative to social situation and impact, whose complexity may often be beyond the comprehension of those not involved in the immediate social circle. (The importance of 'ba' or 'frame' in Japanese social structure will be discussed in greater detail in Chapter 5.) Thus the popular Japanese adage; 'even a thief may be 30 percent right' can be understood.

Appreciating the circumstances of a given situation and the morality that is formed accordingly to factors contained in the situation, in the Japanese context, the Western style of judgement based on a single, unchanging moral code is difficult to reconcile. 'The Anglo-American compulsion for a court trial that determines one party to be guilty and the other innocent is in remarkable contrast to the Japanese ideal that mutual apology and compromise be attained between parties before the conflict attracts public attention'[4] (p. 42). North Americans involved in a (rare) physical altercation on a Japanese commuter train may find it incredible that even though the 'other guy had started it', both parties involved in the conflict are made to share the blame as well as the penalties involved. So, instead of a single transcendent moral code or truth from which all things in the universe can be judged, a cosmology void of such perception, that places humans on a horizontal plane with deities and non-humans, we get a socially relativistic perspective of phenomena. Everything 'depends' on a 'case-by-case' basis.

Morality in this interpretation is socially anchored, based on 'social relativism' involving what is widely known as 'situationalism' or 'situation ethic'. Hamaguchi[8] characterised the Japanese normative orientation a 'particularism-situationalism'. He agrees with Kato[9] in sensing that even universalistic ideas like 'bachi' (heaven's punishment) or 'inen' (karma) seem particularistic in the Japanese social context. Bachi is based on 'the causal law applying to a particular group' (for example, family). It can refer to the punishment meted to members of a group that produced a rule-breaker. Popular still, is the belief that deviance by an ancestor results in the misfortune of a descendent, and wrongdoing by a parent leads to, for example, the deformity of a child. Vestiges of such causal beliefs about disablement lurk in the background of the experiences and self-images of rehabilitation patients. The most negative aspect of disability not being centred on loss of functional performance but rather on the social consequences of the illness, disease or injury.

The subject of Japanese 'guilt' seems inseparable from social relationships and is yet another illustration of a morality directly tied to the social. Takeo Doi[10] believed that 'guilt takes its sharpest form for Japanese when the guilt is generated from the awareness that one might possibly betray the social group one belongs to' (p. 49). When the individual feels he has done something wrong against his or her social group, in spite of the trust the group is imagined to hold for him or her, guilt reaches its maximum. Contrast this with the basis for guilt experience among many socialised into Western life – that guilt reaches its zenith when one has realised that an internally held moral standard has been betrayed. 'You are only betraying yourself (and your morals)' can be a strong statement of indictment by another when one has done something 'immoral'.

Japanese situationalism viewed from the Western monotheistic, individualistic moral vantage is understandably viewed pejoratively. Variability of self, especially with the tendency towards adjusting oneself to an external social context, is likely to be read as a negatively regarded attribute. Such 'other' oriented behaviour is seen as a sign of weakness and synonymous with inscrutability or unreliability. However, it needs to be stressed that once social bonds and obligations to others are established and internalised, the actor is likely to show enormous persistence and rigidity, regardless of fluctuations and changes in the surrounding social. Examination of behaviours among members of Japanese traditional institutions, such as Yakuza (Japanese organised crime networks) or even the fellowship of physicians associated with a university medical faculty, will likely yield such a pattern of rigidity.

There are also parallels between the social relativism tied to the East Asian cosmological myth and aspects of authoritative structure. Alien to interactional relativism is the idea of a single God-like figure who monopolises authority over the whole society. The image of a divine leader, an absolute ruler, or a tyrant who serves as prime mover in secular society is, according to Lebra[4], a product of unilateral determinism. The leader-figure in Japanese institutions, who is socially interdependent, takes on a different function than the tyrant leader or dictator who rules with absolute authority. Often he is merely a figurehead who must rely on the industry of those who are bound to him through mutual obligation.

Although this will be discussed more thoroughly in the next chapter, hierarchy in Japanese society is constructed differently than in other societies. The 'amayakaseru-amae' dichotomy, roughly translated as 'give and take' and which can be observed in typical Japanese vertically structured relationships, ensures that the authority holder is no more autonomous than those who are subject to his or her leadership. A parallel might be seen in how the components of human being are constructed in Western and Japanese cultures. The phenomenon of transcendence can be applied to conceptions of the human body in the West in which the head (containing the brain) symbolically assumes elevated, directive status over the rest of the body. There is a historical tendency to separate a person into mind and body, or into a godly half and a beastly half, and try to subjugate later to the former. This conception of the person is different in Japanese cultures. Rather than a separation, they seem rather to accept a person's whole existence as a balanced, natural unity.

Cosmology, Humans and Nature

Parallels between transcendence of 'mind over matter' and Western man's conceptualisation and attitude towards the environment can be observed in the popular Western notion that the environment must be conquered and controlled. Examples were seen in Chapter 3 in Gustfason's[11] writings about Western religion and attitudes towards nature and the environment. Owing to a cosmology that interweaves self, society, deities and nature into the same tight unity, the Japanese view of nature in relation to the self differs remarkably to the popular Western view. Japanese naturalism is far from either the recognition of nature as independent of human beings, or belief in the subjection of nature to the power of God and man. Rather, the essence of Japanese naturalism seems to lie in an appreciation of the interaction and affinity between humans and nature[4]. It would be expected to be less rationally oriented and void of any individual motives for desiring to 'control' the environment. If Japanese occupational therapists were to develop a conceptual model of occupation or occupational therapy in which humans, their interpretation of agency and their relationship to nature were elucidated, we might expect to see some semblance of this interplay of the importance of nature and humans.

Augustin Berque[12], a French scholar with a long standing interest in Japanese society, agrees in the viewpoint that, whereas the modern Western view of 'self' and environment are seen in opposing terms, to the Japanese they are seen as interactive; the self is constructed in a way in which it melds with the environment by identifying with patterns of nature which are, nonetheless, also culturally constructed. Berque suggests that 'there is a link between the way the Japanese (or indeed people of any society) perceive nature and space, and the way they interact with each other, that is, the way Japanese "self" is defined within its social context' (p. 98). To make his point on this matter, Berque chose to expound on Watsuji's account of Fudo[13], which was regarded to be controversial by its exposition of Japanese uniqueness with the concept of 'Fudosei' (climaticity). Watsuji was perhaps attempting to, with his account, coin a spatial equivalent to the temporal concept of history (rekishisei). His account, like so many others, demonstrates a strong tendency or affinity that the Japanese demonstrate towards nature.

The literature on these matters supports the view that European and Western cultures have tended to give the subject a stable, central, or even transcendent position. The effect is a defining one in which the self is clearly discernable from the surrounding environs. Japanese culture, on the other hand, tends to give the subject a relative position. The effect is one of 'blurring' where the self is less discernable from its surroundings – be it people or the environment. Japanese scholarly works certainly have supported this view of humans in relation to self, society and nature. Kitaro Nishida[14] has written to stress 'basho' (place) and Motoki Tokieda[15] has written in the past to stress the importance of 'bamen'. Yujiro Nakajima[16] is also notable, among many others, to have explored a logic which would be based on the identity of the predicate and not that of the subject. There are numerous other examples of Japanese emphasis on 'process' rather than emphasis on self. One case in point is the traditional 'haiku'. Often the subject or person in the haiku is indefinite while the focus is on the predicate or ambience of the surroundings. That could be a sound, a feeling, or aspects of the natural environment.

The blurring of self in the environment often can also be observed on the grammatical level. 'Samui!' (literally translated as 'cold!') uttered by a Japanese, and the Westerner uttering 'it's cold!' each express their condition in relation to the environmental condition. In the case of the Westerner, the environment is given a separate status with the ascription of a proper pronoun – 'it'. In the case of the Japanese utterance, to a non-Japanese person, it would be difficult to determine whether it was the subject or whether it was the environment that felt cold. Berque[12] asks whether the environment is subjectivised or on the contrary whether the subject is 'environmentalised' or contextualised (p. 96). If we could for a moment take away our rational tendencies to determine which one it is, we could probably imagine better how the Japanese naturally construct their realities concerning self melded with environment in an inseparable way.

Blurring of the self, society and nature can be observed in a variety of other ways. Berque[12] suggests that it can be seen in the organisation of space: 'the Japanese tend to de-center, or displace, the subject's integrating point of view. Unitary perspectives and dominant orientations are not preferred' (p. 99). Roland Barthes[17], in *Empire of Signs*, presents a case for such 'blurring' in the form of Japanese cities. Geometric patterns, rectangular axes running north-south, east-west are largely missing in most Japanese cities. Such rational prerogatives for efficiency and logic, which are the norm in the West, seem to be largely shunned when Japanese cities are studied from aerial photographs. Kyoto and Sapporo are rare cases of such city street designs but these were apparently imported models. Japanese tendencies in this regard appear to favour topological and proximity organisation. Another consideration, when pondering the rationale for such topographic outcomes, is the general temporal orientation of people living in a naturalistic paradigm. An orientation that does not prioritise rationalism blunts the usual future orientation, favouring 'here and now' existence.

The Structure and Sensation of Time

Rational Western views of time tend to look at the possibilities of future outcomes (goals, objectives, dreams, etc.) and logically and meaningfully tie what is being done in the 'here and now' to those objectives. Unilateral determinism demands that we challenge the opposing environment and control our circumstances as much as possible to attain the goals we have constructed ahead of us into the future. The same values and temporal orientation exists in Western occupational therapy practice where we interpret matters of health, disability and client problems on a more individual centred and rational plane. Japanese occupational therapists and their clients may, to the contrary, appreciate more the process of rehabilitation itself over driving practices which aim to yield the right future outcomes. Occupational therapists looking increasingly to evidence-based practice (EBP) as a form of *best practice*, should understand the fundamental issues of time sensation and use in regard to evidence driven outcome ideals and know that people abiding in different world views may be disadvantaged.

Western cultures have striven to give the subject a pre-eminent status. As was opined earlier, this tendency eventually brought forth modern scientific objectivity as an abstraction of the subject from an objectified environment. The traditional Japanese view on individual and environment, which was presented earlier as parts of an inseparable whole, would question the whole notion of an individual agent on a distinctly separate environment.

For the purpose of considering 'occupation' or agency in the *Japanese* social context, several concepts which serve to describe larger (macro) characteristics of Japanese social structure have been selected for this discussion. Where possible, since this elaboration is primarily concerned with *Japanese* constructions of occupational therapy, Japanese sources are favoured over Western conceptualisations and explanations of the Japanese social. These descriptors include but are not limited to the 'Agrarian-Equestrian' societal archetype of Watanabe Shoichi[18] and *'tate-shakai no ningen kankei'* (human relations in a vertically structured society) by Chie Nakane[5]. Descriptions of horizontal social indexing using the concepts of *uchi* and *soto* (inside and outside), *tatemae* and *honne* by Doi Takeo[19], Hendry[20] and Lebra[4], *Jibun-Seken-Tanin* by Doi Takeo[19] are also visited and given due attention. Finally, the concept of *habatsu*, as described and explained by Lebra[4], Chie Nakane[5] and many others, will be reviewed and critically re-examined.

Agrarian Social Beginnings? The Primacy of Nature in Japanese Narratives of Daily Living

Descriptions of Japanese social structure tied to agrarian community social structure are not a rarity in the literature. A substantial portion of *Nihonjinron*, publications which offer theories of 'Japanese-ness' by a variety of academics, journalists and amateur intellectuals[20], is devoted to explaining some seemingly unique aspect of Japanese social structure or cultural attribute to elements of nature.

The use of Watanabe's[18] equestrian (Western)–agrarian (Japanese) archetype is not to be confused with similar archetypes found in *Nihonjinron* literature which favour a more causative relationship between nature and being to advance the notion that the Japanese are a unique (and therefore perhaps a superior) civilisation. Watanabe offers nothing more than a description, or rather a metaphorical dichotomy/dualism that organises observable differences between Japanese and Western (perhaps especially American) behavioural and societal patterns. Watanabe's main postulate, that Japanese society is exemplified by the traditional agrarian village while Western (primarily American) societies are typified by the nomadic way of life, holds more than casual appeal because of its simplicity and use of familiar anecdotes. For these reasons, Watanabe's archetype demonstrates substantial explanatory power in its descriptions of Japanese social patterns, rationales for such patterns and predictability of Japanese patterns of social behaviour. Perhaps most importantly, Watanabe's offering is compelling because he offers his description of Japanese social structure from a native Japanese frame of reference, without going so far as to make causative statements of the origins of such social structure and phenomena.

The Peasant Soul of Japan: Insights into Japanese Views on Occupation

In *The Peasant Soul of Japan*[18], Watanabe attempts to 'propose a theory, of the Japanese Don Peasant as a clue to reading the psychology and behaviour of the Japanese'. He introduces his argument by suggesting that the Japanese have emerged through centuries of agrarian subsistence – a lifestyle that fuses humans to nature and the soil and the cooperative demands of such living necessitates a collectivist social tendency. Subsisting on what the land can produce is arduous work and tilling the soil of a large patch of land requires the organised cooperative work of many. 'Nature giveth and Nature taketh away', it is commonly said, and so the soil supports life and provides security but other natural elements can wreak havoc. As long as everyone does their share of work, there is not much to fear, except for occasional natural catastrophes such as flood, earthquakes and typhoons. Exceptional ability or material wealth does not count for much in regard to status in such a community. On the contrary, such exceptional attributes could draw the envy of others in the community and threaten the harmony that is deemed to be so important to everyone's productivity and survival.

Watanabe asserts throughout his narrative that the ultimate concern of every member of the agrarian village, and therefore most members of Japanese society, is 'security'. The notion of security as a universal concern among Japanese people conjures up thoughts of 'amae' theory in which Doi[21] posits that at the root of every person is a natural yearning to 'draw close' to another … to be enveloped in the warm, protective security of one's mother's arms. The need for security can also be seen in Lebra's[4] postulate that 'belonging' represents the ethos of the Japanese.

In such a group structure, what individuals put their hands to does not need to make rational sense (to the self), nor does the plan of action need to be the most creative or efficient. Personal achievement and self-actualisation are also secondary, if not altogether inconsequential concerns. As long as the collective can remain, and even perhaps prosper, and that everyone has a share in the produce is all that really matters. Harmony, between self and others, and between self and nature are the cornerstones of such security, and members of Japanese collectives will often go to great lengths to contribute towards its achievement.

Watanabe uses the nomadic (or 'mounted bandits, e.g. Genghis Khan and the Tartars) hunter-gatherer prototype, to symbolise the psychology and behaviour patterns of Westerners, and to form a backdrop for comparison in his dichotomous narrative. The image constructed for this prototype stands in dramatic contrast to the description of the peaceful, stable (mundane) lifestyle of the peasant. In the dichotomy, unlike the depiction of the Japanese agrarian collective, Western nomads/mounted bandits are cast as rationally oriented beings who have everything but a stable, calm and secure existence. Subsistence means moving to follow the wandering supply. The focus is on 'tomorrow' and what needs to be done 'today' in order to ensure survival and achievement in the future. Rather than stability, change is normal and one's routine changes with alterations in the surrounding environment. In such a lifestyle, to sit still can mean stagnation in growth and at worst it can spell death. Personal ability, talent, etc., become necessities and are supported and encouraged to grow.

Watanabe also used the prototypical image of successful warrior (namely Genghis Khan, p. 13) to depict the character of Westerners, as well as using historical anecdotes of events in the Second World War as a backdrop to demonstrate differences in the two social patterns. In war, not much matters but the outcome. Therefore, such qualities like efficiency, effectiveness, innovation, speed and creativity, become the hallmark descriptors of the mounted bandit, and the leader of such a group is the one who embodies these qualities.

On Spirituality and Regard for the Land

Japanese cosmology and religion both feature strong metaphorical relations with nature and the soil. In his attempt to convey the modal sentiment of affinity that Japanese purportedly hold for their land, Watanabe begins with a quote from a known unidentified professor of Japanese literature:

> Man's real happiness lies in knowing that he uses the same privy his parents, grandparents and ancestors used, and that his sons and grandsons will use too. Our parents were raised by their parents; by eating rice and vegetables fertilized by their own excrement we live on the excrement of our parents in turn … we can say our own bodies exist as a result of the circulation of the excrement of our fore-fathers, or, as we would say now, its recycling. Our fore-fathers' excrement went into this Japanese soil which produced the rice which our parents ate[18] (p. 25).

Many Japanese who were born around the time of the Second World War can still remember the common ritual of saving human waste, or 'night soil' as a precious commodity which could be used in farming, or sold for cash. According to Watanabe; 'Human waste seems to be valued by a race of people intimately tied to the soil' (p. 25).

Man's fundamental ties to the land and his ancestry are enacted through the eternal cycle of ingesting the bounty of produce from the land, and returning nutrient and soil matter back into the soil through one's excrement. An agrarian people who cleave to the land purportedly find security in it. They are more apt to do so, according to Watanabe, because in times of peace it is the gods and not men who threaten their safety. 'They pray to the gods, they offer sacrifices, and they purify their bodies' (p. 34). When catastrophe hits, the common response is resignation. 'There's nothing to be done ultimately, other than to be resigned, because of damages inflicted by something which is not human' (p. 34).

The author also uses the example of Japanese believing it is important to return the remains of loved ones (such as bones) from foreign places back to Japan, to convey the spiritual quality that Japanese attribute to the land. This can be witnessed even to this day in regular forays by Japanese people to the Pacific war battlefields of the Philippines and other islands, on missions to find and return the bones of relatives to Japanese soil. 'So for the Japanese the whole of Japan seems a holy land' (p. 32). And so it is 'sweet to be buried in the earth of Japan – that feeling is everywhere, even up to the present time'.

> In the country villages in particular, where people use the same privy as their ancestors … there is the feeling of inner security. However poor you may be, if you are born on this earth and raise your children on it, you are immortal. The most fundamental thing in the spiritual structure of the peasant people is this feeling of security (p. 32).

Western 'nomadic' people have transferred their source of security from the land onto their capable leaders. For without commitment to a fixed place, security is conspicuously linked with human ability. In the world of 'occupation' one does not perceive the land to be a part of one's being or necessarily a source of life. The shift of power from nature to human self seems to have occurred with man's transcendence. Nature as an important basis to Western narratives on life and being, as stated in Chapter 3, seems to have disappeared. In Western life, land, like other elements of the environment is not perceived nor socially constructed as such. Land is an entity to be subdued, utilised, occupied and altered according to one's need.

On Leadership

In an agrarian society, where life is lived peacefully, according to Watanabe, great leaders are not really needed.

> You may be a bit senile, you may be a bit paralytic, but if you have (what it takes to maintain harmony) you are more than adequate as a village leader. It does not matter how old you may be, or how palsied, you will preserve the harmony of the village even better because you will not be an entity of anyone's envy (p. 38).

In the agrarian village, Watanabe stresses that there is no great difference between people of differing intellect or ability, provided they do the farm work of the village.

> In a peasant society, even differences in physical strength which are obvious at a glance can be disregarded, provided no special disease is involved. By the same token, we flatter ourselves that the same thing applies to what cannot be seen with a naked eye, like intellectual power (p. 36).

> Prototypical leaders of such agrarian collectives need not be people of great personal talent or ability. Such attributes would only serve to draw the attention and envy of others (and possibly erode harmony). The leader should 'have a willingness to chat to people, to be kind, to be a good listener in awkward situations, to be generous and open-handed' (p. 38).

Nakane[5] also discusses the qualities required for leadership and such arrangements, and she points out that the ability to inspire loyalty is more important than personal merit. Indeed, such a system works rather well if the leader has some weakness and he is obliged to rely on the support of his underlings in some respects. A good leader is also expected to know and respect feelings of his subordinates. This is consistent with Doi's[5] theory of *amae*, in which it is the duty of people in a higher status rank to help and look after subordinates who indulge them. There is a difference here concerning superiority based on weakness and dependency, such as in Japanese leadership, and superiority based directly on merit.

In an equestrian society, a prerequisite of existence itself is to have a suitable leader. The equestrian lifestyle is based on seizing opportunities in a competitive world where the swift and smart exert their advantages. Blessings are taken from others; not received or bestowed from the collective. In the values of equestrian society there is all the difference in the world between the man with a big strong body who can run fast, whose eyes are sharp and his hearing is good, and the dull-witted man who is weak, cowardly and short-sighted. Genghis Khan embodied the prototypical equestrian leader. A shrewd tactician, swift in attack and ruthless in disposing of his enemies, Khan inspired the loyalty of his followers. For who would not place their trust in his leadership? As long as Genghis Khan's armies were involved in their aggressive sweeping conquests, there was less fear, greater feelings of security. The quintessential leader in the Western sense is a figure who has achieved the pinnacle of a system that is based on 'selection' or merit.

On Work Ethic (Agency and Occupation)

Despite other Japanese scholars' acknowledgements of hierarchical social indexing in Japanese society, Watanabe stresses that in an agrarian society like Japan's, despite some differences in levels of wealth, there is a pervasive feeling of equality which makes people vulnerable to envy. 'So we have problems such like "if my neighbour built a barn with a fence, I take offence and feel like I should have the same, too" '(p. 38). Here, I will augment Watanabe's anecdote with another anecdote from Japan.

Upon enduring several cold nights working late in his office at the (Japanese) university, a professor decided that he would purchase a space heater using his personal research funds. The research project he was working on would warrant another week of similar working hours. Since such projects would lead to publication in foreign journals and that such exposure would have some benefit to his university's productivity, the professor decided to ask permission from his university's administrative director to purchase a personal heating unit. The professor's request was flatly denied and when he persisted with a need for an explanation, he was told that the biggest concern was that if he were to acquire such an appliance, all of the other professors would want one too. His immediate (rational) thought was that surely the other professors were not children and could probably decide for themselves whether they needed one or not. The professor left the administrator's office frustrated but mindful that such personal requests, at a university of all places, could not be supported for the sake of social harmony in the institution.

It may be an interesting point of contrast, from a Japanese *agrarian* social perspective, to see that Westerners tend to think that they have what they have because they have 'earned' it. If there's no difference in efficiency between neighbours, though, it is not unnatural to feel resentment if the neighbour's property has a barn and your own house is in a miserable state. Watanabe states that this is another stark feature of an agrarian society. This social tendency – for people to want to be the same and have the same material possessions – persists to the present day and that these values and social tendencies have their origins, according to Watanabe, in the countryside of Japan.

> You cannot have peace of mind until you believe you have proved you are fully the equal of your neighbor, by doing whatever your neighbor does: when he reorganizes his house you do the same as quickly as you can. If you go into the countryside today, you can see in any one village a number of quite splendid houses of similar type. If someone has a house built with the gable-board, the next man who builds after him has built the same. If he has a pond made, the next one also has a pond. If he buys a chandelier, the next one buys a chandelier. And so on (p. 37).

This simple kind of imitation cannot have occurred in the past, because peasants were too poor. But these days, people in the countryside are comparatively rich, which makes it more possible than the past to see these tendencies clearly. Kuwayama[22] probably agrees with Watanabe on this point. His study of the acquisitions of farming machines by farmers of Niike, a farming village in Okayama Prefecture in Western Japan, despite not needing a new machine in particular, would seem to concur. Salesmen, apparently, are well aware of this in Japan. 'If you can get one man to buy even a high-priced consumer product, then it is easy selling the rest. This is how Japan's domestic electronics industry became a world leader. Also, people living in apartment blocks in cities behave in the same way' (p. 38).

Vestiges of this tendency can also be observed on a grander scale when examining the speed and propensity with which Japanese scholars in the health sciences have copied, translated and imported, without prior critical examination and alteration, theoretical material from the West. Why have there been virtually no conceptual models of occupational therapy from Japan, until now? Western counterparts are initially flattered, that foreign nationals would want to emulate them, but may eventually wonder why the Japanese cannot originate or innovate their own ways of thinking. Japanese people may wonder why Westerners apply such pressure (for Japanese to innovate and emerge their own epistemology based on their own contextual needs). After all, they are merely observing materials and ideas that have gained prominence in the West and merely want to follow the same themselves – like a good neighbour.

On Personal Attributes and Advancement

Respect for harmony and respect for ability, do indeed seem to be in inverse proportion to one another in the Japanese context. As a Japanese national, Watanabe believes that his is 'a society in which ability is often regarded as a hindrance ... we value only the preservation of harmony, and neglect ability'. Watanabe believes this to be a real problem and a major factor that led to Japan's defeat in the Second World War. Watanabe contends that the pattern should be recognisable anywhere in Japan. That invariable pattern purportedly is one in which a group of 'inefficient' men have risen to the summit of their factions on the merit of age (seniority). The inadequacies are not merely attributed to eroded physical and cognitive capacity but also to the fact that they have probably been socialised and trained over the years in a milieu that works towards and operates within conditions of social harmony. 'Men who came top in the military academy examinations, and carried out their peace-time duty faultlessly, (rose to their respective leadership posts but) proved to be inadequate at a time when the real enemy was attacking' (p. 56).

At the deepest layer of consciousness in an agrarian society, according to Watanabe, is the feeling of security. And this preoccupation is nurtured and reinforced by the whole social-cultural system. To illustrate this principle, Watanabe uses anecdotes about Japanese government bureaucrats and the process of socialisation within official institutions, which epitomise the utmost in the idealism of 'security'. Traditional Japanese organisations, like government ministries, represent large organisations that hold the image of utmost stability. Watanabe claims that upon gaining entrance into a job with a government ministry:

> career bureaucrats are convinced that they are all equal, in the same way that every farmer thinks that he has the same ability as his neighbour. So if the usual order of things is followed, they are promoted in chronological sequence. Those of lower rank need not be deferential to those higher up since, however candidly they express themselves, their promotion is guaranteed by seniority (p. 48).

So what we have, in effect, in Japanese social institutions by agrarian values and principles, in regard to mechanisms for status acquisition, is a preference for seniority over individual ability or achievement.

Once the 'selection principle' is introduced, where privilege is apportioned according to individual production and achievement, guaranteed promotion based on seniority diminishes. The idea of step-by-step ascension in the social ranks based on individual merit, as reflected in descriptions like the Protestant Work Ethic[23], helps to reify for Westerners the philosophical bedrock that supports the construct of 'occupation'. When Westerners state that occupation represents 'purposeful behaviour', they are implying that agency is applied with rational conviction and interpreted as such. What would happen to the interpretation of occupation if societal rules were changed and the merit attributed to individual effort and ability were nullified? To put it another way, what would happen to Westerners if they were informed that social status or one's rank in the company was to be decided, not on effort, competition or ability, but rather purely on seniority (and perhaps who they were connected to)? Watanabe seems to state it well, when he opines that 'in the world of mounted bandits, there can be no objection to the selection principle because the difference between efficiency and inefficiency is crystal-clear' (p. 27). It can be the difference between life and death.

In the Japanese social context, distinguishing between people solely on attribute may be a difficult endeavour. For one thing, it may be too *rational*, and may not reflect the usual contextual construction of reality. Watanabe would explain that considering persons on the basis of attribute introduces the chance of envy and that envy may lead to disharmony and destruction of the collective sense of security. Nakane[5] might agree as she points out that disparity of attribute in a particular group is usually countered by an emotional approach to overcome it:

> This emotional approach is facilitated by continual human contact of the kind that can often intrude on those human relations which belong to the completely private and personal sphere. Consequently, the power and influence of the group not only affects and enters into the individual's actions; it alters even his ideas and ways of thinking. Individual autonomy is minimized. When this happens, the point where group or public life ends and where private life begins no longer can be distinguished. There are those who perceive this as a danger, and encroachment on their dignity as individuals; on the other hand, others feel safer in total group-consciousness. There seems little doubt the latter group is in the majority. Their sphere of living is usually concentrated solely within the village community or the place of work. The Japanese regularly talk about their homes and love affairs of co-workers; marriage within the village community or place of work is prevalent; family frequently participates in company pleasure trips. The provision of company housing, a regular practice among Japan's leading enterprises, is a good case in point (p. 9).

Japanese occupational scientists and scholars should ponder the contextual interpretations of the concept of 'occupation'. In a social context bounded by values, beliefs and norms associated with individual agency, *occupation* takes on a special meaning and forms an essential concept in the definition of one's *being*. In Japanese social collectives, how is 'occupation' interpreted, especially if individual aspirations are deemed secondary to collective aspirations, which according to Watanabe and other Japanese scholars, are ultimately driven by values that emphasise harmony and security over ability and achievement?

A thought that points to the allure of Watanabe's assertion is that at the soul of every Japanese person lies the heart of the peasant.

REFERENCES

1 US Census Bureau. Report WP/98: World Population Profile. Washington, DC: US Government Printing Office; 1998

2 Iwama M. The issue is ... toward culturally relevant epistemologies in occupational therapy. American Journal of Occupational Therapy 2003; 57(5):582–588

3 Bellah R. Beyond Belief: Essays on Religion in a Post Traditional World. New York: Harper & Row; 1991

4 Lebra TS. Japanese Patterns of Behavior. Honolulu: University of Hawaii Press; 1976

5 Nakane C. Tate shakai no ningen kankei [Human Relations in a Vertical Society]. Tokyo: Kodansha; 1970

6 Pelzel JC. Human Nature in the Japanese Myths. In: Craig AM, Donald H (eds), Personality in Japanese History. Shively, Berkeley and Los Angeles: University of California Press; 1970

7 Haga Y. Kokuminsei juron [Ten attributes of Japanese national character]. In: Hisamatsu S (ed.), Meiji bungaku zenshu [Collected Literature of the Meiji Era], vol. 44. Tokyo: Chikuma Shobo; 1968

8 Hamaguchi E. Nihon-rashisa no sai-hakken [The Rediscovery of Japanese-ness]. Tokyo: Nihon Keizai Shinbunsha; 1977

9 Kato H (ed.) Nihon bunka ron [Essays on Japanese Culture]. Tokyo: Tokuma Shoten; 1966

10 Doi T. The Anatomy of Dependence. Tokyo: Kodansha International; 1973

11 Gustafson JM. Man and Nature: A Cross-Cultural Perspective. Bangkok: Chulalongkorn University Press; 1993

12 Berque A. Identification of the self in relation to the environment. In: Rosenberger N (ed.), Japanese Sense of Self. Cambridge: Cambridge University Press; 1992; 93–104

13 Watsuji T. Fudo. Ningengaku-teki kosatsu [Climate: An Essay in the Study of People]. Tokyo: Iwanami Shoten; 1935

14 Nishida K. Hataraku mono kara miru mono e [From Working Beings to Seeing Beings] (discussed in Nakamura 1983)

15 Tokieda, M. Kokugaku genron [Contemporary Theories of Japanese Language]. Tokyo: Iwanami Shoten; 1941

16 Nakajima Y. Basho/topos. Tokyo: Kobundo; 1989

17 Barthes R. Empire of Signs. Richard Howard, trans. New York: Hill and Wang; 1982

18 Watanabe S. The Peasant Soul of Japan. New York: St Martin's; 1980

[19] Doi T. The Anatomy of Self: The Individual Versus Society. Tokyo: Kodansha International; 1985

[20] Hendry J. Understanding Japanese Society, 2nd edn. London: Routledge; 1987

[21] Doi T. Amae no kozo [The Anatomy of Dependence]. Tokyo: Kobundo; 1971 (in Japanese)

[22] Kuwayama T. The reference other orientation. In: Rosenberger N (ed.), Japanese Sense of Self. Cambridge: Cambridge University Press; 1992; 121–151

[23] Weber M. The Protestant Ethic and the Spirit of Capitalism. London: Allen and Unwin; 1904–5 (1976)

CHAPTER 5

Context and Theory

Cultural Antecedents of the Kawa Model Part 2

心

Much has been stated, both in this book and in the social scientific literature, to describe Japanese people as being collective oriented. This could be an exercise of semantics as many people in Western societies could also describe themselves as being similarly collective oriented. It is when juxtapositions and comparisons along two similarly framed phenomena are performed that we gain a better sense of the contexts and conditions around a particular label or description made of *the other*. Like the realisation of what a vacation means after toiling in a very arduous and uninteresting job, having a foil for reflection makes for a more interesting comparison. From the vantage of a more individual orientation, Japanese people may come across as more group oriented or collective driven. And similarly, from a vantage of Japanese common social experiences that appears to value belonging, interdependence and group harmony, Western peoples may come across as being individualistic, egocentric and self-assured. This approach of juxtaposition and cross-cultural comparison is continued in this chapter for the purpose of elucidating the link between culture and theory. The social context that gave rise to the Kawa model is further examined.

In this second part of the section on the cultural antecedents to the Kawa model, the attention now shifts to the internal structure of the Japanese collective by examining the popular postulates of vertical and horizontal social indexing. If Japanese do perceive themselves in collectives, then what are the mechanisms by which the collective is sustained and along what patterns are they formed? Once again the attention stays on gaining insight into the relationship between cultural context and social theory. In particular, the aim is to clarify how theory is linked and therefore limited to the contexts from which the particular model has emerged. Consequently, the therapist might ask how a particular theory or model is linked to the contexts in and people for which the model is intended.

Very few scholars who study Japanese social structure would disagree with descriptions in the social sciences literature that Japanese society has realised its own unique form of social hierarchy. This hierarchy differs from other known forms along both rules for incumbency and dynamics within and between each vertically indexed level. Unlike the Hindu caste systems of South Asia for example, present Japanese status ranks are not fixed, and differ relative to situation and place. Historically, it is known that in the pre-Meiji era, Japanese society was divided into four clearly defined classes: samurai, peasants, artisans and merchants. People remained in their own classes and were expected to continue living and working (and socialising) and marrying within their same classes. And consistent with Watanabe's[1] postulate, hierarchical ranks often have less to do with personal abilities, talents, or kinship than they do with factors like seniority and social connections.

There is little doubt, both in the literature and in direct observation of Japanese social relations, including analyses of language and communication patterns, that hierarchical differences affect interaction between Japanese people in their everyday lives. According to Hendry[2] and others[3,4,5], most Japanese would experience some difficulty in knowing how to behave unless one can place the other surrounding people in a hierarchical order in relation to oneself. The process of indexing oneself in relation to others differs between Western and Japanese social contexts. Whereas in the West, one might evaluate self and the other in terms of personal attributes and remarkable accomplishments, most mature Japanese people will often examine age, seniority in the group and each individual's affiliation with other prominent people or institutions in order to index self to social environment. The common ritual of exchanging business cards between individuals upon first meeting, presented in the beginning of Chapter 3, is a good example of this prominent social tendency. By examining the card of another, one can place the other in some frame of reference; the kind of (reputable) organisation each belongs to and their rank within their respective frames. The evaluation made in that instance will immediately take effect in each one's behaviour towards the other – how low one should bow and what level of speech to reflect the level of respect accorded to the other. Like the critical importance placed on indexing one's behaviour towards the other, it is also as difficult to engage in proper conversation with another without determining the appropriate level of communication. Perhaps part of the awkwardness that Japanese people feel about conversing with complete strangers is the lack of clear indexing between parties.

If two people of the same age have joined an organisation, such as a company, at the same time, and one had graduated from a top ranked institution like Tokyo University (Todai) while the other graduated from a lesser known institution, the Todai graduate may likely assume a higher rung in the social ladder of a particular group. As will be discussed further on in this chapter, Nakane[3] contends that truly equal status in relations between two Japanese people is virtually impossible, and that Japanese are far more content with social relations on a vertical gradation rather than a horizontal, egalitarian one. Thus Western concepts of *democracy, equal rights* and even *independence* to a certain extent are difficult to conceive. Differences in status as a social norm in the Japanese social context also throws into confusion such imported concepts in health care circles, based on the assumption of egalitarian value, as *patient confidentiality, informed consent* and *client-centred practice*.

Hierarchy in Japanese History

Historians will attest to vestiges of hierarchy in the social structure of Japanese civilisation over the past millennium. Hendry[2] provides a synopsis of the historical record and evidence of status consciousness among the inhabitants of the Japanese archipelago in her book, *Understanding Japanese Society*:

There have been declared differences of status in Japan since at least as far back as the tomb … evidence remains to testify to the material ways in which these differences were marked. Since the emergence of a dominant Imperial family, with an apparently unbroken lineage to the present-day, there has always been some kind of nobility set apart from the common people, even if its practical role has gone through several changes. The Imperial family illustrates a special case of the general principle that lines of demarcation are based on membership in the family order, a common means of distinction which may well go back further. It certainly seems likely that such acquired status has been important throughout the historical period, although it is important to remember that this is not always based on kin connections (p. 77).

There is also some evidence to corroborate Watanabe's[1] assertions presented in the previous chapter that *agrarian* styles of cooperative governance (structured in a hierarchy largely determined along inherited status) prevailed during peaceful, stable eras, giving way to *equestrian* styles of governance and its characteristic status structure determined on individual merit. In varying degrees throughout Japanese history, it has also been possible to achieve status both by individual or cooperative effort. The early warring periods were marked by competition for dominance between groups or factions; competition which had been repeated again and again at various times throughout the subsequent years. Between the periods of conflict, though, lay relatively stable periods marked by people placing greater emphasis on inherited status[2]. The periods marked by wholesale conflict and political instability appear to be transitional, leaving periods of stability (and therefore the agrarian pattern) the normal state of affairs.

The issue of transitions (particularly transcendence) between groups, whether earned or inherited, may have significant bearing regarding the social construction of 'occupation'. Ideas of occupation in the West, where the concept originated, is constructed on the assumption that will and effort, combined with necessary resources, allow one to acquire material and status. Whether it be explained by the Protestant work ethic, Marxist economic theory or some other social postulate, Western ideas about the meaning of agency is based on people fundamentally guided by rational motives. It represents a world view that enables and empowers the individual to live rationally, as if one can, through agency, directly effect change within both one's self and in society. When placed within a social context where effort and merit are not the means by which people earn material or social status, the interpretation of 'occupation' and 'agency' becomes skewed. Inheritance, karma, the will of the collective and other mechanisms that lie outside of the 'self' become the determinants for material and social change. Models that explain agency, empowerment and achievement, steeped in rational, self-deterministic, Western ideals, may be misplaced when attempting to apply them into the Japanese social context.

Ie Structure

The Japanese household structure, referred to as 'ie', figures significantly in the context of Japanese collective life. While examining historical evidence of hierarchy in Japanese social relations, some attention should be paid to the traditional concept of 'ie' (translated into English as 'family' or 'household'. However, like other concepts considered cross-culturally, the term holds implications of meaning beyond these translated terms.) Scholars like Nakane[3] speculate that the seemingly firmly rooted, latent group consciousness pervading Japanese society can be traced back to the institution of *ie*. It has been suggested, but often contested by social scientists, that *ie* represents a remnant of Japanese feudal moral precepts of collectives that are stratified on a vertical plane. Nakane states that:

> the principles of Japanese social group structure can be seen clearly portrayed in the household (*ie*) structure. The concept of this traditional household institution still persists in the various group identities which are termed *uchi*, a colloquial form of *ie* (p. 8).

General consensus though, among critics, is that the *ie* institution is eroding under the pressure of modernisation in the post-war years.

The nature and structure of the *ie* institution is remarkable in its fundamental differences to kinship bound institutions of family as defined in other Asian countries and the West.

> The Japanese family system differs from that of the Chinese system, where family ethics are always based on relationships between particular individuals such as Father and, brothers and sisters, parent and child, husband and wife, while in Japan they are always based on the collective group-members of the household, not on relationships between individuals[3] (p. 9).

The formation of social groups on the basis of fixed frames, and not kinship, remains characteristic of Japanese social structure. The common saying, 'the sibling is the beginning of the stranger' is an accurate reflection of Japanese values towards ideas about kinship.

> An unmarried sibling who lives in another household is considered a kind of outsider. Towards such kin, duties and obligations are limited to the level of the seasonal exchange of greetings and presents, attendance at wedding and funeral ceremonies and the minimum help in case of accident or poverty (p. 9).

Nakane has further commented that the shift away from kinship forming the basic unit of the social has been compensated in this modern phase by a greater emphasis and importance attributed to a 'personalized relation to a corporate group based on work, in which the major aspects of social and economic life are involved' (p. 9). Once again, the classification of self-in-relation-to-group in terms of 'frame' and 'attribute' is put forward. These concepts are expanded upon in greater emphasis in the next section. The discussion thus far underscores the complexity of Japanese collectives and brings into question the validity and relevance of contemporary ideals of occupation as developed by occupational therapists and scholars situated in the West.

Tateshakai No Ningen Kankei: Human Relations in a Vertically Structured Society

No recent reference in the literature addressing Japanese social structure seems to be complete without some attention given to the work of Japanese social anthropologist Chie Nakane, in her book[3] *Tateshakai no ningen kankei* [Human Relations in a Vertical Society]. The name Nakane seems at times to ring synonymous with any discussion regarding the hierarchical structure of Japanese social relations. Nakane's postulates and the main principles of those postulates are presented briefly in this chapter and discussed in relation to their implications for the construction of occupation and occupational therapy in Japan.

Forming the basis to Nakane's theory is the concept of 'ba' or 'frame' as the author has chosen to conceptualise it in English.

> Frame may be a locality, an institution or a particular relationship which binds a set of individuals in one group: in all cases it indicates a criterion which sets a boundary and gives a common basis to a set of individuals who are located or involved in it (p. 1).

Takie Sugiyama Lebra[4] had described Japanese patterns of behaviour to be based on social relativism or 'situation', and this situation is, I believe, consistent with Nakane's 'frame'. The situation or frame is comprised of space, imaginary or real, and all who are involved in it. The frame, whether it be a discrete physical place in time, and institution, or a relationship between people, comprises the criterion point from which truth of matters are interpreted and reality constructed. Unlike Western interpretations of reality and truth, based on universal morals or on ultimate truths, Japanese people appear to have traditionally held a more naturalistic world view which is ascribed to situational ethics and *flexible* truths.

'Attribute' is another important concept in Nakane's theory and is used to indicate those (people or matters) that are associated to a common 'frame' or 'ba'. 'Attributes', thus, are named or associated to, or rather 'belong' to, a given frame. Several individuals who are employed by the same frame, Company A for example, may each be considered an attribute of Company A. This is not to be confused with Western interpretations of the concept of attribute, which is usually understood to refer to some special qualities that define an individual from another. Nakane's conceptualisation of the term differs from the common Western in that her 'attribute' is not interpreted to be universal as it might be in the West. By universal attribute, I am referring to traits and characteristics that an individual holds which will not change in its interpretation going from group to group or from situation to situation. Physical attributes such as hair colour, body type or fashion preferences and non-physical attributes such as interests and temperament or character are typical examples. The tendency of the Japanese to stress situational position in a particular frame, rather than universal attribute, can be seen in the following example: when the Japanese person faces the outside (confronts another person) and fixes some position to himself socially he is inclined to give precedence to institution over type of occupation (p. 2). In exchanging business cards or when introducing oneself over the telephone, it is a common tendency to give the frame first, followed by the attributional detail. The name of the company or institution is given first followed by one's name. Following this, one's actual occupation or role within the organisation might be offered. Consider how these exchanges play out normally in your own contexts. Do you typically introduce yourself before stating the name of the organisation you represent? In Japan, it is almost always organisation or group identity first, followed by personal identity. A typical introduction of self over the telephone may be as follows: 'Hello, this is the University of Tokyo's Department of Biology's, assistant professor, Yamada...'

> The listener would rather hear first about the connection with B publishing group or S company; that he is a journalist or printer, engineer or office worker is of secondary importance. When a man says he is from X Television one may imagine him to be a producer or cameraman, though he may in fact be a chauffeur. In-group identification, a frame such as a company or association is of primary importance; the attribute of the individual is a secondary matter. The same tendency is to be found among intellectuals: among university graduates, but what matters most, and functions the strongest socially, is not whether a man holds or does not hold a PhD, but rather from which university he graduated. Thus the criterion by which Japanese classify individuals socially tends to be that of particular institution, rather than universal attribute. Such group consciousness and orientation fosters the strength of an institution and institutional unit (such as school or company) and is in fact the basis to Japanese social organization ... (Nakane, p. 3).

Contrast this emphasis on frame with Western patterns of status evaluation, which tends to prefer the individual's universal attributes over frame. For the Westerner, where one works or which institute one has graduated from is, of course, not without significant meaning. A professor at a leading university receives his due respect, but the professor in all likelihood has risen to such status through the merit system. Ultimately, the more rationally driven Western world view is more apt to value what an individual is personally capable of and what results he or she has achieved over time. Status is evidence of achievement in Western spheres of social experience. And achievement comes from competence and effort. 'Occupation' in the Western sense, where the concept originated, is enveloped in this ideology; of emphasising attribute over frame. If Nakane's postulates of Japanese social structure, with its emphasis of frame over personal attribute are valid, then the interpretation of the central construct of occupational therapy, occupation, becomes problematic.

In the 'kaisha', or company, where many Japanese are employed, this perspective of 'frame' and 'attribute' takes on special meaning. Unlike in the West, where the employer represents one of many aspects or ties in daily life that one may have, to the Japanese person, it symbolises the expression of group consciousness. Earlier in this book, the discussion involving the conceptualisation of 'self' in the contexts of individual and collective society, it was postulated that the collective oriented Japanese is not only strongly influenced by his or her 'seken', but also derive their sense of identity from their social frames. Western occupational therapy theories conceptualise the *self* as a distinct, self-deterministic entity who 'occupies' time and space through purposeful (rational) agency. In these depictions, it was noted earlier that productivity (work), leisure and self-maintenance comprised the domains of occupational performance. In the West, individuals have a sense that they, themselves, determine their affiliations and choose when, how, and where they will use their time and effort. If Nakane is correct in her summation of the primary importance of *frame*, then it may mean that a reverse dynamic to the Western might be evident in the Japanese context. That is, the employer (frame), and its corresponding social collective, time, activities, etc., chooses the individual. The Japanese individual, then, is seen more by Westerners to be passive recipients of social roles, status and responsibility. After all, one merely becomes an attribute to the more important, all determining frame. It is no wonder, then, that Japanese students and practitioners of occupational therapy experience such difficulty grasping the concept of 'occupation' as Western occupational therapists discourse it.

Considerations for Role Theory

Traditional role theories[6,7,8] are appropriately challenged when critically examined from within Japanese social contexts of collectives structured hierarchically. In particular, social psychological assumptions about interactions in which people come to acquire their roles (rather than describing the place of these roles in the social structure) are called into question. In the Western experience, where self is constructed to be situated at the centre of the universe and self-determinism reigns supreme, role taking (people taking the role of the other) and role making (people constructing their own roles) are common behaviour patterns that can be witnessed in everyday life. However, if identity and being, for people existing in collectivist social contexts are not perceived to be situated or contained within oneself but rather more broadly to include others in its definition, the dynamic of role taking loses a great deal of its explanatory power. Japanese people may, less than their Western counterparts, be seen to target a particular social status role and move rationally to assume it. Rather, roles are status positions or stations in particular frames that the collective, or someone higher in the system representing it, bestows upon the individual. Role acquisition then may be greater influenced by extraneous factors such as age, seniority and social connections, rather than interest, will and resources within one's disposal[9].

'Doing, being, becoming'[10] is a well-known phrase in recent years in occupational therapy that defines the beneficial outcomes associated with 'occupation' or agency. The phrase gathers all of the tacit beliefs that Westerners more or less hold to be true about the essentiality of agency in defining the Western sense of being. The concepts in the phrase are purposefully aligned, directionally, and reflect values attached to agency, existential meaning and to human potential. Many Westerners believe in the 'right' to be whatever one chooses to be, and that achieving one's dream is simply a matter of having the will (drive) and applying one's God-given abilities through agency. Deciding upon a career direction may simply be a matter of yielding to one's own interests and applying an adequate amount of effort over time. It is a rational process whereby one sets appropriate goals and sets a plan to work methodically towards them. Difficulties along the path need to be confronted and cleared out of the way. From this perspective, roles are, by and large, positions in society to be 'taken' (through a rational application of agency).

For the Japanese, agency is not necessarily a means to define one's being, nor is it a tangible means to acquire or construct a role. The social frame 'bestows' or allocates a role to an individual and once that role is accepted and assumed, the role duties (or 'yakume' in the Japanese language) are played or carried out. Role-defined duties are taken assiduously, as if one's life depended on it. Perhaps this is because one's *yakume* is evidence of one's connection to a particular collective (frame). And if a Japanese person's identity and definition of 'self' are strongly tied to collectives, or frames, one's allocated role has an extraordinary effect upon one's sense of identity and construction of 'self'. As an attribute to a frame, tasks that are apportioned as part of one's role need not make rational sense or have tangible meaning. One need not even know how the task in question fits into the bigger picture. What matters is that one has a role and as a result has been given a task that affirms one's connection to the collective. The pre-eminent task is to carry out that task to completion as expected by the collective. Lebra's[4] postulate, that 'belonging' represents the social ethos of the Japanese, certainly rings affirmatively here. In contrast, if the Japanese were to use a variation of Wilcock's[10] expression to rationalise the situation of roles vis-à-vis agency (doing), then 'becoming, being, and doing' might be more fitting. Role, which is arguably tied to a Japanese person's sense of being and 'belonging, which is perceived to be granted (by the collective), determines and applies meaning to the execution of tasks.

Whereas a Westerner may feel discouraged or deflated when meaningful tasks (occupation) are suddenly taken away, a Japanese person may feel similarly so when they are separated or barred from their social group (frame). It is well reported yearly, in the Japanese media, that children often commit suicide as a result of 'ijime'. (Roughly translated as 'bullying', but in the Japanese social context, holds a differing pattern of repercussion. This form of bullying includes ostracism by the collective, and in the context of collective societies, where 'identity' and 'self' are intensively tied to the collective, the effect can be psychologically devastating, often resulting in suicide.)

Residuals of this social pattern can be seen in the Japanese workplace, especially in various relations between the employee and the employer. Nakane offers that the relationship between employee and employer cannot be explained in simple contractual terms. Rather the employee is enveloped ('marugake' is a familiar Japanese term often used when discussing the total commitment of the employee to his employer. It means to 'be completely enveloped') by the employer in the spirit of the common saying, 'the enterprise is the people' (p. 15) and it is mutually assumed that the 'total man' is being employed. This tie between enterprise and employee, or rather between frame and attribute, is an all-encompassing one and its strength may be correlated to the strength of marital ties between husband and wife. This may be difficult for a non-Japanese person to comprehend, for in the West, the lines of vocation and personal life are normally clearly delineated. The tendency to appear to be more loyal to the employer than to your own family or relatives would be considered abnormal and likely be looked upon by others unfavourably.

Role tasks will, in all probability, be tackled with a sense of fervor and personal responsibility. Failure or mistakes are largely unconscionable and the resulting disparity in feeling is the sense that one was not able to carry out their 'yakume' dependably, thus letting down everyone in the collective. Here it is appropriate to recall from the previous chapter the differences in cosmologies and world views and subsequent effects on relational being. The Eastern cosmological myth lacks a rigid monotheistic belief system yielding an arrangement of morals and truths that are flexible and dependent on context. Unlike the modal rational Westerner, who tacitly believes that the world and self are constructed on an ultimate truth, the modal Japanese person is more susceptible to construct the world and self relative to social contexts. Rather than basing one's actions on, or interpreting other's actions from, a singular set of universal moral precepts, the Japanese are subject to basing and interpreting agency on amorphous moral precepts which crystallise when set in a particular social context (frame). The common reply of; 'case-by-case', to questions put to a Japanese person about how they feel about moral dilemmas such as infanticide or sexual harassment, may not necessarily be so outlandish, when considered in this socially relativistic context.

The Structure of Frame or 'Ba'

As mentioned throughout this chapter, Nakane's main thesis is that generally, Japanese groups share a common structure and internal organisation in which members are bound together vertically in a delicately ordered gradation. Two simple diagrams graphically portray Nakane's postulates. First, Figure 5.1 shows an inverted 'V' to show how a group based on hierarchical relationships are structured. The second figure (Figure 5.2) portrays an expansion of the former structure to illustrate how relationships form layers. Each person in the system occupies a rung in the grade so that no one else shares the exact same status in the vertical gradation. One more evident feature is that while there is always someone likely to be situated above you (sempai), there will likely be someone situated below you (kohai). So delicately ordered is this hierarchy that two individuals of the same age and sharing the legacy of having graduated as classmates at a prestigious university, will mutually settle accordingly into a gradation where one will be ranked higher than the other. Once rank is established, behaviour and language can be adjusted and set accordingly.

Westerners should take note that the criteria used for such ranking often have little to do with individual talent or ability. Depending upon the institution or group, the criteria often take seniority into account (years of service, or even years since a certain qualifying examination was taken). Ranking according to seniority rather than on personal merit is regarded by many Japanese people

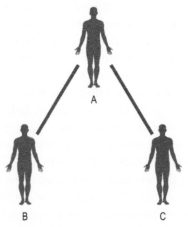

Figure 5.1 Graphic depiction of Nakane's inverted 'V' principle of Japanese social organisation patterns.

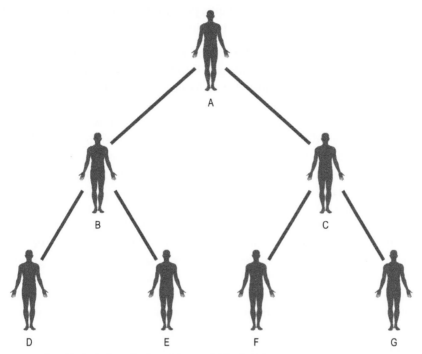

Figure 5.2 Graphic depiction of Nakane's inverted 'V' principle, expanded to illustrate how consistent the same relational structure can be layered.

to be simpler and more stable, however, such a system is also regarded to be more rigid. There is only one ranking arrangement and no individual member, no matter what his or her rank, can make any changes to it. Barring catastrophe or some outside disturbance, which can result in destruction of order or disintegration of the group, the hierarchical structure will in all likelihood persist.

When groups coalesce into a rigid hierarchical structure with tacit rules of behaviour and responsibilities that correlate with rank or position within the hierarchy, they are often referred to as 'habatsu' or *factions*. Traditionally such *habatsu* have often been observed in familiar social institutions such as in political parties, the military (and self-defence forces), gangs and entertainment guilds. There, such terms of ranking such as 'sempai' and 'kohai' can be replaced by the more familial 'oyabun', and 'kobun'. Though the rigidity of structure in such factions seems extraordinary, Nakane's writings would indicate that the *habatsu* structure is merely an extension of the basic model of group structure in Japanese society. In the same way that individual behaviour and sense of self might be strongly determined by one's rank and relationship to others in a given 'frame', individual behaviour and social influence in *habatsu* perhaps are more obviously manifested. Anecdotal evidence would point out that groups that function well over a long period of time have a greater chance of evolving into *habatsu* status. The strength of human relations, based on implicit value placed on loyalty, perhaps tends to grow over time and find its expression in the form of such rigid factions.

In institutions like companies, schools, and public offices, the Japanese person can easily find his or her world divided into three defined categories; *Sempai* (seniors), *Kohai* (underlings) and *Dohryo* (colleagues). Chie Nakane[11] contends that a person who has no awareness of his or her relative rank to others is not able to speak or even sit and eat with the others. He will not know how to act or verbally address others appropriately and thereby risk offending other members or be seen as being someone who is disrespectful of others. In Japanese academic circles, this principle has a profound effect upon the process of scholarly debate and the synthesis of new ideas. In my own experience, at the university where I was employed, the pattern of professors with seniority dominating the discussions while lower ranked research assistants and lecturers remained verbally non-participative was the norm. Furthermore, it is rare for younger Japanese professors to openly disagree with their seniors. One would rather be silent, it seems, than utter flatly negative words such as 'no' or 'I disagree'. This direct influence of hierarchical rank on free expression of individual thought imposes a significant impediment on the academic process. This may be a stark example of how Western scholarly tradition, which is heavily steeped in rationalism, encounters profound limitations when brought into the Japanese social arena. Nakane[11] astutely uncovers this fundamental limitation inherent in vertically graded social structure. 'The premises underlying thesis-antithesis are parity and confrontation on an equal footing which will develop into or permit the possibility of synthesis'. The lack of such experience and ability, coupled with a situational-relative construction of truth, contributes to a dearth of new ideas. For over 35 years, since occupational therapists' inception in Japan, Japanese occupational therapy scholars have yet to develop their own, original, conceptual model of occupational therapy. The evident trend of directly copying and translating theoretical models, including assessment batteries from the West, en masse, will likely continue.

Social structural influences in other realms of health and occupational therapy practice and behaviour can now also be postulated. The first such instance which readily comes to mind can be observed in the dynamic relationship between the client and the health professional. Invariably, the client will come to the hospital or alternative clinical setting with a specific need. That need is essentially to have a health problem or difficulty rectified. Most clients will voluntarily/automatically assume the lower status designated to those who seek the indulgence of others, in relation to the health professional[12]. Vestiges of Parson's[7] conceptualisation of the 'sick role' in its similarities can be seen in this relationship. Though hierarchical structure can still be observed in the culture of biomedicine in the West, its existence on the backdrop of Western egalitarian societal norms gives it a different expression in comparison to the Japanese. Biomedicine's inherent hierarchical structure transfers well onto the social backdrop of Japanese hierarchical social structure. Because studies verifying this difference were few in number, I interviewed several Japanese physicians who had experience of treating foreigners in their Japanese practices. These physicians unanimously remarked that (Western) foreigners question and make more inquiries about their treatments than their Japanese counterparts. The rationale being drawn here is that Westerners bring with them a sense of right which places the relationship between health professional and client on a more equal footing. Thus, the client is more apt to assert their right to question and agree to the interventions suggested by the professional. If one is not satisfied with a given opinion or procedure, a second opinion with another health professional can be readily exercised. The issues of patient confidentiality and informed consent (before any invasive procedure is performed) also hinge on these egalitarian social structural traits.

For the Japanese patient, assuming the role of patient (attribute) in the hospital under Doctor so-and-so's care (frame) and performing the tasks befitting the role, including tacitly held obligations, is seen to be essential to the smooth operation of the medical process. Western expectations for 'client-centred practice'[13] in which the patient or client is expected to take the primary role in the rehabilitation process, by shaping treatment goals according to one's own outcome goals and expectations, would be extremely difficult to implement in the Japanese context. Expecting a person who has come with the expectation to be a model patient and receive instructions passively and obediently would undoubtedly require a colossal shift in perceived roles and role expectations.

Challenges to Nakane's 'Tate Shakai' Model

At this juncture, some mention should be made about the structure of Japanese hierarchical social structure. On initial examination of such descriptions of the hierarchy, one might be inclined to assume that this pattern is pervasive through all social relations. However, it must be said that Japanese *situational* ethics and relativism also are readily observable in most social instances. Further on in this chapter, the concepts of *uchi* and *soto* (inside and outside) are addressed in greater detail, and it should be mentioned here that there is also an 'inside' and 'outside' quality to such social hierarchies. Formal status positions and social roles may be subsumed by individuals in any given context but behind the formality that is shown outwardly, there may be, in actuality, different degrees of differences (negligible to substantial) behind the scenes. Politicians perhaps present convenient examples of this pattern. The general citizenship are not lost on this however, as they all, sharing the same ethic *know*, perhaps expect and in many cases *accept* there to be something else or a variation of what has been so neatly presented on the outside. In Western nations, the Prime Minister or President wields a considerable amount of power and is held accountable by the collective through the process of suffrage. If he or she is found to be dishonest, or not acting on the will of the people, the leadership will likely change with the next election. In Japanese politics, the political leader may assume a strong image befitting the mandate of his office. However, in reality, he may not actually wield any real power. The differences between outward and inward expressions of status and power are not always found in this pattern in which the vicarious character is weaker than what is seen on the outside.

An anecdotal example of such can be found in the well-known folklore 'Uchi Benke'. The main character in this amusing Japanese story, Benke, is a fellow who is seen as a weak individual in public but who turns into a powerful tyrant in his own home. Like Jekyll and Hyde, are the dramatic swings between personality profiles but what differs in Benke's personality is that changes are conditional to situation (frame or place-dependent). Well-known social scientists such as Benedict[14] and Dumont[15], have also remarked about the important distinction between the fixed position one occupies according to the rules of hierarchy, and the quite different degree of dominance or power that one may wield behind the scenes. Although inner and outer characteristics are quite separate, invariably the inner (vicarious) is given no right to violate the outer public image. Multiple examples can be witnessed in Japan through all levels of formal institutions and in everyday life. Such socially relativistic social ethics and behaviour have confused and often annoyed uninformed visitors from the West, who assume that the Japanese, like themselves, abide by a universal set of moral precepts that are not contingent on situation or frame.

Chie Nakane offered her compelling anecdotal postulates without providing much empirical evidence. For her lack of scientific analyses, her postulates have come under considerable criticism. However, the basic tenets of her postulates cannot be easily refuted, as many Japanese will concur that these structural depictions are both real and readily observable in daily life. For harnessing certain behavioural patterns readily observable among most Japanese and major institutions, 'Tate shakai no ningen kanke' appears to possess considerable explanatory power for describing the root of Japanese social behaviour patterns. On the other hand, the model has been criticised for attempting to be too all embracing, and stereotypical, among other things. Hendry[2] had observed that Nakane's book (*Japanese Society*) has no references or bibliographies to support her postulates. Nakane's arguments utilise examples that rely on anecdotes instead of empirical studies. Hendry notes that Nakane's descriptions are sometimes slightly distorted to emphasise the point, and occasionally the generalised statements are very sweeping. Nevertheless, the principle outlined is very pervasive, and the author is able to draw on her experiences in India, Europe and the USA to compare its operations in practice with the different social hierarchical principles found elsewhere. She reiterates, for example, the way the Japanese vertical principle differs from that underlying a caste or class system in India, and examines some of the consequences of these differences. Nakane's structural analysis, despite its generalising effect is still a useful framework to assist scholars interested in Japan to conceptualise and study Japanese society and patterns of agency.

Horizontal Indexing: *Uchi* and *Soto*

In discussing certain prominent macro social characteristics of Japanese society, Japanese 'collectivism' has been likened metaphorically to the traditional peasant village structure[1], which is hierarchically stratified. In order to gain a greater appreciation of Japanese group structure and how certain micro social tendencies might influence and share structural characteristics on a grander, macro scale, the discussion requires expansion into the interpersonal indexing realm. In the ensuing discussion attention is turned to yet another evident form of social indexing in Japanese society.

This additional conceptualisation of social structure is horizontally posited and evidence pointing towards its existence can be seen and heard in such ubiquitous and dichotomous terms as *uchi* and *soto, omote* and *ura*, and, *tatemae* and *honne* (Figure 5.3). These and other dyadic terms have been frequently observed and commented on in the social scientific literature on Japan; for example, in situational relativism[4], in political hierarchy[16], in business enterprises[17,18], in health and illness[19], in constructions of 'self'[20] and religion[21].

These vernacular Japanese terms, which can be roughly translated into English as 'inside' and 'outside', 'in front' and 'in the rear' and 'outer display' and 'inner truth', respectively, imply that such dichotomous indices may be part of Japanese people's construction of reality and subsequently how their social worlds are structured and perceived. It may also be significant that

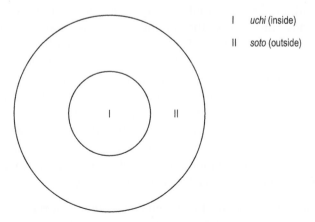

I	*uchi* (inside)
II	*soto* (outside)

Figure 5.3 Doi's model of 'uchi' and 'soto' (adapted with permission from Kuwayama T. in Rosenberger N (ed.), Japanese Sense of Self, 1992, p.145, Cambridge University Press).

during common reference to these paired concepts, the terms that denote outside, or the public domain, almost always supersede the term denoting the commonly hidden inner or private realm. This should come as no surprise for those who support Nakane's postulates of frame over attribute. In such collective societies like the Japanese, the social group's aspirations are frequently placed ahead of the individual's aspirations. The group's aspirations are often seen as public knowledge while individual concerns are often relegated to the hidden 'private' realm. Once again, we are afforded glimpses of the special social-cultural contexts in which 'occupation' is to be defined and expressed.

Somehow occupation, or purposeful doing, has to be reconciled within the tension between 'inside' and 'outside'. Others' actions and behaviours must be filtered through a set of social conventions, which separate to a certain extent, the intention of the other's actions into inside (basic, personal intent) and outside (deliberate, outer or public intent). By the same token, one may process their actions through a similar filter of 'inside' and 'outside' intentions. Situations vary in time and space according to Lebra[4], and the 'Japanese distinguish one situation from another according to the economy of inside and outside'. Lebra further iterates that inside means internal and private, while 'outside' means the opposite – out, outside, external, and public. She proceeds further by explaining that Japanese people are known to differentiate their behaviour by whether the situation is determined as inside (personal and secret) or outside (open to the public). The boundaries between inside and outside seem to be variable according to situation and appreciated at different levels. Inside and outside may refer to a distinction within an individual, one's family, a group of friends, an institution, a community or internationally. For example, an individual may carefully separate his private inner feelings from his outer public expression. On a more macro level, one might be concerned about not allowing an embarrassing incident of national proportion to be viewed by other nations. Members of a university faculty or other organisations like a manufacturing firm, for example, will conscientiously limit any information that might taint its reputation – either interdepartmentally or to the outside. The inside–outside conscientiousness, which also can be similarly observed in the West, are especially prominent in the Japanese social context giving the common locution about 'face' particular credence. In a collectively oriented society, where one's 'face' and position is strongly determined by the surrounding social, due attention is paid to presentation. Failure to do so may elicit profound negative consequences to one's daily life and future chances. In this way, it can be argued that certain aspects of agency or 'occupation', as it is often referred to in the West, is conceived of and shaped by social and cultural contexts.

The situational variability of 'inside-outside' conjures strong images of the naturalistic mores of the East Asian cosmological myth[22], whereby unlike the Western cosmology, where a defined singular set of morals stand at the root of behavioural production and interpretation, a diffuse, varied and pliable system of morals may prevail. Should varied moral structure be not critically contingent upon a singular transcendent deity but rather upon other human beings and elements of the social, then Lebra's[4] postulates concerning the 'prime mover' would appear to coincide with this particular analysis. The main source or element that controls or gives impetus to human behaviour, according to Lebra, tends to be located inside the self in Westerners and outside the self (social environment) in Japanese.

While pondering Lebra's postulate that the social ethos of Japan is 'belonging', we are able to imagine how differently the core concept of occupational therapy – occupation – may be conceived from the Japanese social experience. While Western conceptions of occupation are anchored to agency (or 'doing'), I will add a postulate that Japanese conceptions of doing are anchored to the social. Likewise, whereas independence serves as evidence of a child reaching maturity in the West, having the social skills to interpret and navigate through the relativistic Japanese social context, including inside-outside, and the 'vertical principle', serves as evidence of a 'well-adjusted' Japanese adult.

Horizontal Social Structure

The basic unit to social groups can be conceptualised as 'self' in the individualist, Western sense or as 'individual in relation to the group' in the group-referenced Japanese sense. The individual and society are conceptualised differently according to two different frames of experience. One reflects a world view and construction of the social on transcendent, monotheistic and rational beliefs and value patterns while the other reflects a world view and social construction on naturalistic, pluralistic, situational belief and value patterns. Kuwayama[23], in his study of the 'reference other' orientation in a farming village of Okayama prefecture, Japan, posits that there are three distinct categories of *others* in Japanese social relations which are concentrically related to the self (*jibun*) as the centre: *mawari*, *hito* and *seken*. Kuwayama has translated these concepts as 'immediate reference others', 'generalised reference others', and 'reference society', respectively. These terms are illustrated in Kuwayama's diagram which has been reproduced in Figure 5.4. What is interesting to note is that as one becomes more removed in distance from each of these groups, their influence on shaping the self (*jibun*) does not necessarily weaken. A case in point can be observed in everyday Japanese life in which the middle concentric layer, defined as 'hito' (generalised referenced others), which is arguably the most abstract entity in Kuwayama's depiction, can strongly influence individual conviction and agency. 'Hito ni warawareru' – 'you will be the subject of people's laughter' – is the example offered in Kuwayama's text, to illustrate how Japanese parents might appeal to the imagined reactions of others to a child's questionable behaviour, in order to

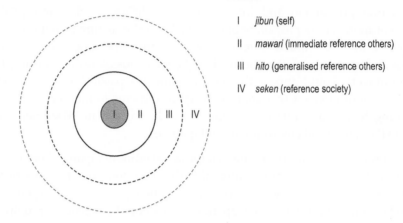

I	*jibun* (self)
II	*mawari* (immediate reference others)
III	*hito* (generalised reference others)
IV	*seken* (reference society)

Figure 5.4 The reference other model. Kuwayama's diagrammatic depiction of 'self', 'mawari', 'hito' and 'seken'.

inhibit it. That is to say, the Japanese child is purposely made aware of and sensitised to others' scrutiny, feelings and opinions[24].

Other Horizontal Indices

The inside-outside dichotomy represented by *uchi* and *soto*, described earlier in this chapter, can also be found metaphorically in other vernacular Japanese expressions. *Honne* (inner truth) and *Tatemae* (outer display); *Ura* (in the rear) and *Omote* (outer presentation); *Mae* (front) and *Ushiro* (back); and *Hara* (abdomen) and *Kuchi* (mouth) are but a few examples of such paired expressions that partly reflect the structure of horizontal indexing in Japanese society.

Tatemae, to the unimpressed Westerner may be taken simply to mean that which is put up like a façade to conceal the real truth of the matter – which is thought to be hidden or held 'close to the chest'. In this way, *tatemae* and *honne* like its other similar dyadic counterparts might be interpreted to stand for two distinctly exclusive entities. Taken this way, *tatemae* may be assessed a pejorative meaning in accordance with values which connote such purposely planted exteriors with deceitful intent, while its counterpart has been delegated legitimate status according to its relationship with 'truth'. So strong is this implication that when Westerners especially hear that a piece of information is merely *tatemae* they are apt to assume that it is false and that *honne* represents the 'real truth'. No doubt, many people in Japan have put up *tatemae* in a quest to deceive others but the Japanese may not necessarily judge this social tendency as such. *Tatemae* and *honne* behaviours are, in the context of social collectives, necessary for the sake of fostering harmony in social frames.

In the Japanese construction of reality, each of these dyadic pairs may not be mutually exclusive terms but rather two sides or views of a given reality. Several writers, such as Doi[25] and Lebra[4], have suggested that without one of the paired terms, the other cannot be fully appreciated. Doi has remarked that the 'consciousness in grasping things simultaneously in terms of both their aspects of "omote" and "ura" is especially well-developed in the Japanese language' (p. 24). That is to say that without the *tatemae*, or outward expression, the full understanding of *honne* cannot be appreciated.

> First, consider the etymology of the word tatemae. It is beyond doubt that the '*tatemae*' of tatemae and honne was originally the same word as the word tatemae in Japanese architecture, which means raising the ridge pole. This work was considered to be so important that the owner of the building under construction would treat the master builder and his helpers to a lavish banquet after it was completed. Tatemae is also the word used in the tea ceremony for the formal movements of the host in presenting utensils and serving the tea. In both architecture and the tea ceremony, the tatemae is essential. If the 'tatemae' of tatemae and honne is indeed the same word, it is impossible to believe that it is unimportant[20] (p. 35).

Doi further offers that:

> In short, tatemae and honne always implies the existence of a group of people in its background who assent to it. In contrast to this, honne refers to the fact that the individuals who belong to the group, even while they consent to the tatemae, each have their own motives and opinions that are distinct from it, and that they hold these in its background. In fact, these individual, personal ways of viewing the tatemae in themselves are said to be honne (p. 35).

Similar related meanings can be attached to the other dyadic terms here. One half of the dyad referring to the public expression, the other referring to the private expression. Both terms of a pairing appear to represent two mutually exclusive entities but, in fact, from the Japanese contextual perspective, are merely two aspects of the same truth.

Philosophical Considerations

In the previous chapter, it was suggested that the rational-oriented Westerner is apt to divide his or her world into separate entities. Self in relation to an environment are initially viewed as separate entities. The concentric rings in Figure 5.3 should not be confused with such a rational supposition. For the Japanese, the orientation of self, vis-à-vis the environment, may not be such a rationally separable one. Self or 'jibun' may be imagined to be immersed in the environment inseparably, and not simply set side by side as separate, mutually exclusive entities. Perhaps through this supposition, we can appreciate the influence of transcendental, Cartesian views of 'self' and 'world' which have through the years, in the West, convinced us of a rational, particular structure of self and construction of reality. That Japan and Asia for the most part did not have these influences from ancient times but rather evolved world views from an East Asian version of the cosmological myth[22] (which is not incongruent with the tenets of Mahayana Buddhism and the Confucian system of ethics) would suggest that views of self and environment constructed alternatively to the Western construction are indeed probable.

Western interpretations of *occupation* rely on self and environment as being mutually exclusive entities which become conjoined through agency. Doing, being and belonging had been already offered as an example reflection of this philosophical orientation. If one is imagined to be immersed in the environs and that there is no need to join together that which is already joined (by nature), Japanese people may be strongly reliant on the here and now, rather than towards a rational bent that is future oriented and realised through occupation/agency. If self is conceived to already be a part of the environs (leaving no need to span the two entities through agency), many Japanese people may not construct occupation as a universally fundamental concern like Westerners are apt to do – certainly not as a necessary property of *being* and *belonging*.

Some Problems

Review of the literature reveals an array of vantages on Japanese social indexing which present a series of problems for the social scientist in search of universal standards or principles for analyses. Researchers like myself, who take a position of cultural relativism, will argue that cross-cultural analyses of the social present almost insurmountable difficulties in order to render bias-free outcomes. At the core of the problem lie issues pertaining to construct validity. Do the terms and concepts employed in the analyses hold similar meaning among the research sample, or between researcher and research subject? Just how do concepts that are formed and tied to the local cultural context of meanings hold their meaning – with all of the cultural nuances attached, when transplanted into another profoundly differing context? The transplantation of occupational therapy, which was founded in the West, on Western value patterns, in a Western social context, being transplanted systematically into the Japanese context is one case in point and subsequently forms the subject of this thesis.

An important element to keep note of when we formulate descriptions of social structure and characteristics is that context is shaped by patterns of social experience. In this chapter, the collectivistic conceptualisation of the Japanese has been taken further by discussing its anecdotal similarities to agrarian social organisation, its vertical hierarchical leanings and its inherent horizontal social spacing or indexing. These, coupled with a selection of micro-aspects of the Japanese social described in the next chapter, present a stark contrast to the social milieu from which occupational therapy had emerged.

One other threat to the validity of the social scientific discourse on Japanese society, which is rarely touched upon in the literature, is the biases inherent in the very (Western) concepts utilised as descriptors of Japanese social phenomena. As we shall see in the ensuing next chapter, the English term 'dependency' and its Western interpretations of meaning do not give justice to the Japanese social-contextual derived 'amae'. For dependence is but one aspect of the constellation of meanings surrounding the Japanese concept of *amae*. By the same token, the clear 'un-shifting' Western context-derived concepts used empirically to describe Japanese social phenomena, such as 'hierarchy' or 'index' cannot be relied on universally to hold exact meaning in varying contexts. How do such foreign terms, which in themselves connote 'order', 'logic', and other concepts that suit the rational, unwavering views of modern science, adequately describe or explain a society that has been described by its own scholars as being relativistic, shifting and situational?

At some point, the dialogue among Western scholars considering Japan may need to determine whether the conventional pattern of social scientific enquiry bolstered by Cartesian, rationalistic and monotheistic philosophical and world views can adequately capture and explain Japanese society and its inner dynamics. Failure to do so may inevitably ensure that the distorted interpretations of Japan and Japanese society will continue to amuse Westerners but do very little to benefit Japanese people and explain realities as the Japanese interpret them.

All of these issues and others pertaining to rational analyses of the Japanese social reflect various facets of the same problem. The relational self, situated social order, vertical principle, embedded points of view, and shifting all pose the same general question for the organisation of Japanese self, society, and language use: namely, how can these aspects of context that are particular, situated, embedded – or identified with uniqueness – be identified with general principles, or patterns that transcend context? Perhaps one answer to this question is in the suggestion that particular social contexts cannot be easily identified with general principles nor be described adequately by terms and conventions formed in a different social and cultural context.

Occupational Therapy in the Context of Japanese Social Structure

In earlier sections of this book, the social contexts of the Western hemisphere were presented in an attempt to shed light on the most salient qualities of occupational therapy; a context founded on the basic transcendent value patterns that gave rise to and continues to sustain the spirit of individualism. This was an orientation of thought which undoubtedly supported the emergence of independence, volition and egalitarianism as ideals in Western social life. It was also the ground from which our current ideas about truth had its beginnings. Hobbes, Locke and Descartes founded a tradition of science, which afforded a world view favouring logical, mechanistic ideals. The preference for reason, of finding causative relationships between phenomena – a belief that any phenomenon could be reduced to a set of truths – became a standard by which all things could be judged and interpreted. In the social sciences, the influence of rational thought preferences are virtually inescapable, for they form the very basis of our affirmations of what we believe to be true and credible. The resulting explanatory power of scientific processes has persuaded many scholars to favour rational explanations of social phenomena and lean towards a set of universal theories and models to explain truth and reality for all.

Depending upon how it is viewed, Japan and Japanese society present an array of interpretations; from a culture driven by 'shame'[14], to 'modern industrial miracle' with vestiges of the exotic orient, to modern industrial enigma[26] which has risen to great economic power but lacks clear political purpose and direction. This work, which has decidedly taken a cultural relativistic perspective of Western and Japanese occupational therapies, supports the viewpoints of those few scholars who prefer interpretations of reality as the Japanese might socially construct it. These viewpoints, which postulate that Japanese agency is driven and shaped by distinctively different constellations of common beliefs, value patterns and social norms from those of the West, challenge universal assumptions and conventional (Western) conceptions of 'self', social reality and *occupation*.

From the approach that this work has taken, Japan is presented to have evolved a social structure distinct from others based on differing philo-sophical, religious and historical patterns, as virtually every other distinct society has. In the previous chapter, Watanabe was quoted to have anecdotally likened Japan's society to that of an agrarian, rice-farming community, in contrast to the nomadic mounted bandits typifying Western society; its main feature being the collective orientation towards long-term security rather than short-term and immediate success. The Japanese affinity with nature, as described in the East Asian cosmological myth[22] in the previous chapter was recognisable in Watanabe's anecdotes. In such a lifestyle, in which security is tied to the soil, as long as the seasons dictate what occupations are performed, change is slow to come. In fact, change may be unfavourable as it might upset the natural order of phenomena, the peace and harmony that may follow.

The Cultural Exclusivity of Contemporary Occupational Therapy Theory and Epistemology

In the preceding chapters on world views, the apparent fundamental differences in conception of 'self' vis-à-vis society between Japanese and

Western social structure and *cultures* were explored. Given the suggested, perceivable separation between an omnipotent deity, self, society and nature as a result of transcendence, Western 'selves' have spanned the voids between these separated entities through agency. Through purposeful 'doing' Western individuals have found a way to exert their presence on or 'occupy' their physical and social environs, and in doing so have exercised their God-given 'right' to self-determinism and self-actualisation. How then is the orientation and perceived purpose for 'doing' conceived in a world view that constructs self, society, nature and deities in a common singular, cohesive entity? How does our regard for agency differ in such a non-rational world view? Does one need to act purposefully on the environment in order to 'be'? The universality of popular Western-based notions of humans depicted as 'occupational beings' is challenged and possibly falters on this very factor. Japanese, or other peoples' inability to grasp Western notions and meanings of 'occupation' can be traced back to this fundamental construction of self, society and nature. Western ideas about occupation or 'doing', independence and personal causation are contrasted to Japanese emphases on 'belonging'[4], interdependence and collectivism, including Watanabe's essay on societal archetypes.

The vertical and horizontal organisation and indexing of social relations apparent in the Japanese social context presents yet another profound set of implications on the interpretation and expression of 'occupation'. Coupled with the influence of collectivism on construction of 'self', we can appreciate the prominence of 'ningen kankei' – or human (social) relations – at the core of individual Japanese behaviour and agency. Contrast this to the Western social condition in which individualism, self-determinism and personal causation are permitted and are set in a system of social mores aligned with egalitarian values and an arguably more lenient horizontal index. As Lebra[4] had stated, whereas the 'prime mover' in social agency is situated within the Western individual, the prime mover in the Japanese context is located more outside the individual (and closer to the surrounding social environment). It is not about what 'I want to do and will do', but rather 'How will my existence and subsequent action fit in with the existing social environs?'

Emphases on 'the other' (instead of on 'me') in collective societies, in the framework of a hierarchical social structure, requires occupational therapists to rethink their long held assumptions about role acquisition and role performance. In the egalitarian sense, life roles are conceived as being freely attainable and disposable. Under God, every individual has as much right as the next individual to pursue his or her choice of career and path in life. The importance placed on human agency to determine one's lot in life is observable in such common anecdotes as 'you reap what you sow', and 'God helps those who help themselves'. Life is 'one big race', so to speak, and there is a tacit agreement in Western society that anything is possible given the right measure of personal determination, talent and effort. A poor man's rise to wealth and success through sacrifice and hard work are applauded while lack of success carries an implication that the individual did not try hard enough. In occupational therapy, it was Mary Reilly[27] who affirmed that profession's fundamental bond with these values by stating her canonised quote: 'that man, through the use of his hands, as energized by mind and will, can effect the state of his health' (p. 2). That one can freely pursue one's lot in life, set personal goals and move independently and rationally to *achieve* them, implies that even social roles can be freely pursued and attained.

The construction of self in a rational, individualist sense, as well as role attainment based on merit gives us a view into how disability and well-being are experienced in Western cultural contexts. The celebration of personal agency and individual determinism contributes to the construction of disability – or lack of ability and skill to perform and achieve – as a personal tragedy. By the same token, the pursuit of well-being appears to be tied to matters of personal talent and effort. In this way, occupational therapists need to understand the hidden values and culture in their existing theoretical material, ideology and knowledge systems. In certain contexts, occupational therapy may achieve just the opposite of its well-intentioned aims.

When the prime mover is located outside of the individual and firmly positioned in the surrounding collective, roles can be seen more as something determined and appointed by the social environment rather than of one's own invention. And if Japanese scholars Watanabe and Nakane are correct, your granted social role may have been determined by factors other than talent, self-determination or individual effort. Your role may have been determined by socially determined factors such as your age, who or which institutions you are connected with, and virtues which do not draw the envy of others such as patience and long suffering. Your role may have been significantly affected by loyalties, both to you and to others. Putting it simply, in the West, roles are more apt to be earned through selection on personal attribute and merit, while in collectivist societies like Japan, the dominant social pattern may still be that roles are determined and granted by the collective. Effort is expended towards achieving and maintaining social roles, while in Japanese social life, people may find themselves expending effort because their social roles (determined by the collective) dictate them. In a Japanese cultural context, one might be thoroughly content with this arrangement as having assumed a role in the group may be affirmation of one's status within it. The ensuing sense of satisfaction of having assumed a particular role may not necessarily be in the sense of accomplishment of having achieved that particular social role but rather in having been granted one by the collective group that one is incumbent in, for role acquisition may not be perceived to be a result of one's own making but rather entirely due to the benevolence of the group one is surrounded by. And accepting a role entails the acts of dependency on others (higher in social status) and indulging those who (lower in social status) depend upon you. Depending on others, in Japanese cultural contexts, constitutes a very important occupation.

Occupation is thus set in a profoundly different social context and is apt to take on a peculiar meaning in the Japanese social. Occupation (or 'doing with purpose') may be viewed by Westerners as a means for individuals to gain their sense of being in the world in which they live. By 'doing', social roles can be targeted and rationally acquired. For the Japanese it is postulated here that occupation (interpreted narrowly for this purpose) takes on meaning in the context of the social collective. Instead of conceiving occupation as a means to an end (role, sense of being), occupation may represent the expression of one's being and role in a collective. Whereas Westerners appear to place agency at the centre of their concern, Japanese might prefer 'ningen kankei' (human relation) or Lebra's derivative, 'belonging'[4], as the ethos to their existence.

These few factors presented in this and in previous chapters infer that social structure and culture hold profound influence on the therapeutic relationship and dynamic in occupational therapy. How patients view their own status, health care need, and role in relation with members of the health staff are all profoundly affected by these and other fundamental social factors. Problems that might have been framed as matters of self-efficacy and weakened independent agency by occupational therapists holding a Western perspective might be interpreted by a Japanese therapist as being a broader social problem with 'ningen kankei' (human relations) taken as the most important rehabilitation concern.

In the Japanese social, no two people in a frame are equal in status. There will always be a hierarchical relational structure exerting order in the relationship between therapist and client. Social rank-position will influence what and how one conveys oneself. It is not a mutually exclusive dynamic. The other will respond and receive such communication using the mutually accepted and expected register and behaviour. In this manner, Western 'client-centred' occupational therapy theory and practice may not be possible in the Japanese social context. Both the therapist and patient will most likely experience much difficulty in assuming role-positions and scripts that stand opposite to 'normal' Japanese social convention. (For more on this problem, see Iwama M. Cross-cultural perspectives on client-centered occupational therapy practice; a view from Japan. Occupational Therapy Now 1999 CAOT, Nov/Dec, (4–6).)

There is a broader message here for those who have laboured through these chapters on Japanese social structure and cultural views of reality. The relationship between culture, social context and occupational therapy theory has hopefully been elucidated and made clearer. While the examples used here have been primarily those of Japanese and Western perspectives, occupational therapists reading this material are encouraged to re-examine their own cultural contexts in which they perform occupational therapy. They are implored to use a broader definition of culture, as 'shared spheres of experience and meaning', rather than the individually bound definitions that treat culture as static embodiments like ethnicity and race. A culture may consist of a particular age group, geographical location, religious orientation, sexual orientation, economic status, aboriginal group, job status, etc., any group of people who share common experiences and meanings of such experiences.

The solutions to the problems of incongruence and occupational therapy theory, epistemology and practice being culturally out of sync with the real world of clients are not simple. For occupational therapy to be one of the greatest ideas[27] in the field of medicine, occupational therapists may need to allow the core concepts and processes of occupational therapy to be reconceptualised[28] along the cultural norms of the target group for occupational therapy. In turn, this will require new theoretical materials to be developed and older materials to be adapted. Occupational therapists will need to find better ways to enact client-centred approaches that develop theory and knowledge from the ground up. We need to pay greater attention to practice. New conceptual models and ideas of occupational therapy need to be developed by people who have the most relevant and recent knowledge of the contextual world and circumstances of the client. How client centred are we being if we carry out 'client-centred' approaches that force the client to comply to standard questions and protocols and force the client's narratives into unfamiliar constructs and principles situated in unfamiliar and possibly unsafe contexts of meanings?

REFERENCES

[1] Watanabe S. The Peasant Soul of Japan. New York: St Martin's; 1980

[2] Hendry J. Understanding Japanese Society, 2nd edn. London: Routledge; 1987

[3] Nakane C. Tate shakai no ningen kankei [Human Relations in a Vertical Society]. Tokyo: Kodansha; 1970

[4] Lebra TS. Japanese Patterns of Behavior. Honolulu: University of Hawaii Press; 1976

[5] Doi T. Amae no kozo [The Anatomy of Dependence]. Tokyo: Kobundo; 1971 (in Japanese)

[6] Goffman E. The Presentation of Self in Everyday Life. Garden City: Doubleday; 1959

[7] Parsons T, Shils EA (eds). Toward a General Theory of Action. Cambridge: Harvard University Press; 1951

[8] Mead GH. Mind, Self, and Society. Chicago: University of Chicago Press; 1967

[9] Triandis H. Collectivism vs. individualism: A reconceptualization of a basic concept in cross-cultural social psychology. In: Verma G, Bagley C (eds), Cross-cultural Studies of Personality, Attitudes and Cognition. London: Sage; 1988; 61–95

[10] Wilcock A. Reflections on doing, being, and becoming. Canadian Journal of Occupational Therapy 1998; 65:248–256

[11] Nakane C. Japanese Society. Tokyo: Charles E. Tuttle; 1973

[12] Iwama M. Cross-cultural perspectives on client-centered occupational therapy practice: a view from Japan. Occupational Therapy Now 1999; CAOT, Nov/Dec, 4–6

[13] Law M, Baptiste S, Carswell A, McColl M, Polatajko H, Pollock N. Canadian Occupational Performance Measure, 2nd edn. Toronto: CAOT Publications; 1994

[14] Benedict R. The Chrysanthemum and the Sword: Patterns of Japanese Culture. Boston: Houghton Mifflin; 1946

[15] Dumont L. Essays on Individualism: Modern Ideology in Anthropological Perspectives. Chicago: University of Chicago Press; 1986

[16] Ishida T. Conflict and its accommodation: omote-ura and uchi-soto relations. In: Krauss E, Rohlen T, Steinhoff PG (eds), Conflict in Japan. Honolulu: University of Hawaii Press; 1984

[17] Hamabata MM. Crested Kimono: Power and Love in the Japanese Business Family. Ithaca: Cornell University Press; 1990.

[18] Kondo D. Crafting Selves: Power, Gender, and Discourses of Identity in a Japanese Workplace. Chicago: University of Chicago Press; 1990

[19] Ohnuki-Tierney E. Illness and Culture in Contemporary Japan: An Anthropological View. Cambridge: Cambridge University Press; 1984

[20] Doi T. The Anatomy of Self: The Individual Versus Society. Tokyo: Kodansha International; 1985

[21] Hardacre H. Kurozumikyo and the New Religions of Japan. Princeton: Princeton University Press; 1986

[22] Bellah R. Beyond Belief: Essays on Religion in a Post Traditional World. New York: Harper & Row; 1991

[23] Kuwayama T. The reference other orientation. In: Rosenberger N. (ed.), Japanese Sense of Self. Cambridge: Cambridge University Press; 1992; 121–151

[24] Clancy N. The acquisition of communicative style in Japanese. In: Schieffelin B, Ochs E (eds), Language Socialization Across Cultures. Cambridge: Cambridge University Press; 1986

[25] Doi T. The Anatomy of Dependence. Tokyo: Kodansha International; 1973

[26] Wolferen K van. The Enigma of Japanese Power. Tokyo: C.E. Turtle Company; 1993

[27] Reilly M. Occupational therapy can be one of the great ideas of 20th century medicine. American Journal of Occupational Therapy 1962; 16:1–9

[28] Iwama M. The issue is … toward culturally relevant epistemologies in occupational therapy. American Journal of Occupational Therapy 2003; 57(5):582–588

Raising a New, Culturally Relevant Conceptual Model of Occupational Therapy from Practice

力

How universal and therefore applicable to *other* social-cultural contexts are the ideas, assumptions and theories about human agency and praxis that underlie contemporary ideas of occupational therapy? A survey of the professional literature informing occupational therapy thus far reveals few studies or papers that have critically examined the validity and applicability of Western theoretical models to explain the meaning of *occupation* and occupational therapy in other geographically situated social and cultural contexts. The dearth of original occupational therapy models or attempts to adapt existing conceptual models, which have largely been constructed on middle-Western social and cultural norms, may lead many to presume that the concepts and ideas of occupational therapy are universally applicable and that non-Western occupational therapists and their clients, such as those situated in Japan, do not differ much from their Western counterparts. That occupational therapy's core concepts, theory and epistemology remain primarily informed by one particular world view bounded by social norms and practices germane to Western spheres of experience renders the profession and practice exclusive from a cultural perspective.

What has been asserted throughout this book is the realisation that contemporary theories about human occupation and occupational performance strongly reflect the modal values, beliefs and social norms of the social contexts they were emerged out of. A cursory glance at the structure and concepts of recent conceptual models in the profession reveal a conceptualisation of human *occupation* that is particularly monistic, rational, future oriented and individual focused. Egalitarian social structure and the ideal of independence are also strongly represented. The absence thus far of alternate theory and epistemology in occupational therapy that diverge from these norms may lead many occupational therapists to presume that contemporary ideas about occupational therapy are sufficiently universal and that there is no particular need to expand its social mandate. However, seen from another cultural construction – one like Japan's which has been described at some length in Chapters 3 to 5, as polytheistic, naturalistic, temporally oriented to the 'here and now', collectivist, interdependent, and hierarchical in social structure[1] – occupational therapy can appear to be esoteric and out of touch with others' realities.

This is not to suggest that original and useful theory does not exist in other non-Western cultural contexts. In all likelihood, in the confusion that prevails around how concepts about occupation are interpreted into local contexts of occupational therapy, the clinician situated outside of Western social norms has unwittingly developed some theories of his or her own. That is to say, that current occupational therapy practice outside of *middle*[2] (North) America is not an anomic process where intervention is based on some random process. There are constellations of implicit rules, persistent value patterns and rationales for intervention that occupational therapists use to guide their occupational therapies. These remain to be uncovered, made explicit and available to the contemporary theoretical discourse in occupational therapy.

FN Kerlinger[3] defined theory as 'a set of interrelated constructs, definitions and propositions that present a systematic view of phenomena by specifying relations among variables, with the purpose of explaining or predicting phenomena' (p. 9). It follows, then, that if a theory is valid and reliable, it should help to describe and explain phenomena, predict occupational therapy outcomes, and guide both research and clinical interventions. By Kerlinger's explanation of theory, therapists situated outside of modal Western social contexts indeed have developed and actually use *theory*. They may not regard these cognitions as theories because their comprehensions of *valid theory* in the empirical sense have been symbolically misrepresented by theoretical models transplanted from foreign cultural and social contexts. Unaltered, transplanted models represent constructions of reality that appear to hold less meaning and relevance to their own shared experiences and world views. Embedded in their current clinical patterns of practice and decision-making are the cognitive patterns and templates of order that each therapist finds useful to explain and guide their interventions and actions. Implicit in their interpretations and decisive actions are the essential makings of new, alternative and culturally relevant theories of occupational therapy practice. The tenets of their tacit models may not necessarily be unique and entirely different from those Western models they have adopted. Most likely, these occupational therapists have reconciled their own interpretations of reality, social patterns and systems of values with mainstream Western interpretations of reality, social patterns and systems of values embedded in occupational therapy's philosophies and ideals. Their particular conceptions of occupational therapy, no doubt, have also been strongly influenced by the biomedical frame of reference and its enormous explanatory power that forms the institutional structure in which occupational therapy is practised in many industrialised societies.

A Brief Review of Descriptions of Western Individualism: The Bases of Prevailing Occupational Therapy Theory

Discussions of the differences of peoples' value and belief patterns were put forward in Chapter 3 which involved comparisons of worldviews or cosmologies. The notion of cosmological myths or collectively held views of the universe's construction as fundamental starting points to examining influences on peoples' values and belief patterns was illuminated to compel occupational therapists to understand the possibility of alternate narratives on the meaning of truth, self, society, and nature. Briefly, once again: the remarkable difference between the East Asian cosmological myth and the Western variation of it was stated to be the radical transcendence of an all-powerful God or Truth. This transcendence separated the elements of self, society, nature and deities from their imagined singular tightly bound unity, into graded entities on a continuum. The transcendence of a single omnipotent deity in Western cosmology[4,5] can be viewed to correlate symbolically with the individual's transcendence over others (society) and nature (environment), having been bestowed dominion over these elements by a single omnipotent God (see Figure 3.2).

Whether or not such cosmological myths and particular world views have had any bearing on a given social group's value and belief systems, certain traits or conceptualisations have been raised often in the literature to describe Western individualism. Some of these concepts described the modal Western individual as being *analytic, monotheistic, materialistic* and *rationalistic*. Further to the rationalisation and separations of man and the elements of his universe, the environs were explained to be viewed by Western man as a separate entity placed in opposition to the 'self'.

It was also suggested that ideas on *unilateral determinism*[6], *self-efficacy*[7], and *personal causation*[8] reflected a particular attitude or way of looking at the world in which the individual was compelled to occupy their environs through purposeful action. Thus it was assumed, as Lebra[6] had postulated, that the prime mover for one's actions was located within the individual for the Westerner with the ultimate objective being to gain competence and independence by establishing control over his or her circumstances. In such spheres of experience and meaning, rewards as well as taking responsibilities for performance outcomes become more the domain of the individual than of the surrounding social context (or collectives).

The Western tendency to construct the world in an analytical, particulate manner, which is congruent with a particulate view of self, society and nature, represents an important tenet of occupational therapy philosophy. That problematic tenet is the objectification of 'external' objects as existing separately from the observer. The view of the environment (both social and physical, etc.) seen in opposition to the self (connected through 'occupation') rather than viewing the environment as just one part of the same unified whole, holds profound consequence for whether peoples of other cultures can share the Westerner's interpretation of occupation and its supposed essentiality to *well-being*.

A world view that is constructed along monotheistic, materialistic and analytic interpretations lays a foundation for rationalism. All phenomena, including human agency and praxis can be systematically investigated and explained by some rational logic. In regard to occupation, we might interpret it as 'purposeful behaviour in which we tie certain means to certain ends'. The basing of our *doing* on some objective or purpose, or tying what we do in the present with the past and, perhaps more importantly, the future, is representative of our rationalistic priorities. Human behaviour that lacks purpose or looks to be randomly executed may draw immediate admonition from another to 'come to one's senses' and to 'be rational'. It represents a value-laden, cognitive pattern made possible in a world perceived as structurally ordered and set in motion by certain universal laws. Tying one's action or 'doing', rationally, to some future objective temporally orients the individual towards the future. Often actions are evaluated in regard to how they are linked to past events and future objectives. The current preoccupation with outcome measures and best practice based on evidence is perhaps an extension of this value pattern.

Postulates regarding the congruence between Western world views and occupational therapy theory should be readily evident in occupational therapy theory, particularly those conceptual models that purport to explain human agency and its qualities. Graphic representations of occupational therapy's current conceptual models readily reveal the importance the authors have ascribed to the individual subject by placing him or her in a central, privileged and authoritative position. The narrative on human occupation in these models almost always constructs the central individual as agent, expected to act rationally on the surrounding environment – a separate but encompassing stage upon which occupations are defined and appreciated. The degree to which an individual can *control* his or her life circumstances becomes valued outcome validations for therapeutic goal attainment.

In these Western constructions of well-being is the notion that personal achievement or self-actualisation represent the acme of human strivings and that these ideals are derived through a process of exploration and competence. 'Mastery' of self and the environment (nature) becomes equated with healthy states of being. In this way, occupational therapy conceptual models represent and reify Western ideals of health defined along individualistic and rationalistic proclivities. How appropriate, then, are these depictions of health based on the ideals of individual agency, for a society that abides by a very different social and cultural construction of reality?

We turn then to the work of a group of Japanese occupational therapy clinicians who were not only unable to make sense of these narratives of doing and being but were concerned about the consequences of not knowing what occupational therapy was beyond specific practice forms and skills. How often have therapists in one particular dominant culture encountered difficulties in delivering satisfactory occupational therapy to clients from a different culture? The barriers to understanding common experiences and resolving misunderstanding often go far beyond mere language. Differences in basic world views, reality, values, beliefs and traditions and customs that are thought to influence and drive health behaviours, are often overlooked despite their profound consequences. These same challenges of the cross-cultural competency of therapist and client from different cultures, also prevails in cross-cultural understandings of occupational therapy ideology and theory.

Cross-Cultural Viability of Occupational Therapy Theory

In Chapter 3, the East Asian version of the cosmological myth[4] was described suggesting for example, that there may be a strong tendency among Asian peoples to perceive the world differently from peoples of Western cultures. That description of the Eastern and 'primitive' world view typically placed nature, self and society in a 'closed' tightly integrated whole. Nature, deities, self and society would be viewed and experienced as integrated elements of an inseparable unified whole (see Figure 3.1). There are no social-structural after-effects of a radical transcendence of a single God, single truth or single moral code. Rather than linear ties of loyalty and trust extending (vertically) towards a single deity or universal ideal, they settle into a complex, flexible constellation of (horizontal) human relations. With regard to human behaviour, the *social* (in absence of an omnipotent deity) becomes the entities by which all things are valuated and judged. Persistence of the cosmological myth in Eastern conceptualisations of nature, self and society, compared to the Western transcendent, separated version of it, can be correlated to certain observable social-structural patterns. This world view, for example, may limit the conceptualisation of the centrality of 'self' in the universe as well as deflecting reliance and attribution of accomplishment away from a solitary, centrally situated self.

In the case of Japanese social contexts, such a 'decentralised' conceptualisation of self purportedly permits a 'situation ethic'[6] to determine behaviour whereby the social situation more than the centrally constructed *self*, strongly influences the interpretation, initiation and shape of human agency. And with emphasis placed on horizontal social relations tied to 'frame' in Japanese social experience, a social-focused norm gains prominence over an individual-focused norm where matters pertaining to existentialism and identity are contingent on 'doing'. Thus Lebra's suggestion that the 'prime mover', which is located internally in most Westerners, is seen to be located external to the self in the social 'frame', for the modal Japanese person.

Following this brief discussion on the East Asian version of the cosmological myth and its proclivity for a particular world view that places the social or collective foremost over the individual, a summary, though admittedly brief, on the main descriptors of Japanese social structure prominent in the social scientific literature, was offered. Some of the ideas and concepts applied in descriptions of Japanese social structure and characteristics in Chapters 4 and 5 included the agrarian archetype[9], vertical indexing (*tate shakai*[10]), and horizontal indexing (*uchi, soto; jibun-seken-tanin*[11]) and *amae*[12] – a concept describing the microdynamic of interdependence between superior and subordinate. These concepts were discussed for the sake of surfacing particular aspects of Japanese self, society and nature, which contributed to the social context into which occupational therapy, brought from the West, was being reconciled. These descriptors were presented to give the reader a sense of the social and cultural context for which a new, alternative narrative or model would need to be developed. They provide a rationale for the structure and content of the Kawa/River model of occupational therapy.

A Society's Imagined Affinity for Nature in Life Narratives

A society structured in parallel with the traditional Japanese agrarian community is commonly shared anecdotally in many Japanese social circles to provide an archetype of Japanese social structure and modal behaviour patterns. Shoichi Watanabe's *The Peasant Soul of Japan*[9] was recalled in Chapter 4 of a Japanese person's description of Japanese social structure using the metaphor of an agrarian community. Farming life represents subsistence on the land and the tilling of soil requires the cooperation of many. In this construction of daily living patterns, the Japanese person was typecast in a cooperative relationship with nature and society. Anecdotally, a historical rationale was being given for Japanese people's profound affinity for nature. Seasons and climate dictate the rhythm of tasks and no one person is capable of achieving anything by one's self. It is the soil and nature that bestow life, not some singular, omnipotent and omnipresent God. Nature giveth and nature taketh away. The nature, that provides the bounty that is essential for life, can also remove by natural catastrophes of typhoon, floods and earthquakes. This was more of a representation of the East Asian cosmological myth in Japanese folklore and its expression into the collective consciousness of the Japanese person. Variants of Mahayana Buddhism and Shinto – Japan's national religion – have complemented and reinforced the modal Japanese person's socialised sense of being inseparably embedded in nature.

As in the metaphor of an agrarian community, in which its members must cooperate to produce from the land and ensure survival, rather than values being primarily placed on cultivating individual attribute and capability, they are placed on equality and cultivating group harmony. Further, the *balance* striven for among and between humans and the soil (nature) is a different conceptualisation of *balance* as related by Western occupational therapy theorists like Kielhofner[13]. Western notions of balance with nature are connoted with having sufficient ability to tame and *control* nature. In the realm of Western occupational therapy, the notion of balance of self and the environment can be deconstructed along the concepts related to occupational function seen in the early renditions of the Model of Human Occupation[14,13]; *exploration, competence*, and *achievement*. In the West, it is primarily about *doing*, and subsequent *results*, that form the basis to the conception of human well-being. In Japanese society, *doing* is important but may not mean much when separated from the social context in which it occurs and from which meaning is derived. States of well-being are contingent on human and natural relations. From the collectivist perspective of Japanese scholars like Watanabe[9], exceptional individual attributes can draw the envy of others. The strengthening of such individualism threatens social harmony necessary for collective organisations or community's production and survival. Thus, harmony between self and others and between selves and nature, forms the cornerstones on which 'security', belonging and states of well-being among

Japanese people ultimately rests. The necessity to belong and the persistent drive for harmony form the basis to Japanese 'collectivism'. This form of collectivism is contingent on a world view that diverges from rationalistic views of singular universal truths. It is a view that sees all elements of nature, including humans, as inseparably integrated.

Maintaining and advancing social ideals, theory and knowledge systems that are based on and reified by a relatively narrow world view renders occupational therapy culturally exclusive and limited in its capacity to make a meaningful and positive difference in all peoples' daily lives. In this post-modern era of relativism, a profession like occupational therapy cannot survive and prosper in the global arena if it keeps its cultural myopia and fails to recognise and understand the particular and variable quality of clients' perspectives of being and doing.

Professional Identity Crises: The Impetus for a New Model of Occupational Therapy

Out of a conflict in differing social contexts, between West, where occupational therapy was founded and conceptualised, and Japan, where these social-context rich ideas have been systematically implemented, emerges a funda-mental problem of *meaning*. In the West, culturally appropriate theory has had a profound effect on the profession of occupational therapy. Miller[15] related that theories function to explain, describe and predict phenomena and Western occupational therapists have benefited from culturally appropriate frames of reference that reflect, explain and help to predict outcomes regarding their experiences of *occupation*. By trying to fit theory and assessments based on cultural patterns so remarkably different from those of the Japanese, a pro-fessional crisis was evident. The concepts of imported occupational therapy and theories have been left largely unreconciled to indigenous experiences of reality. They are written in a foreign symbolic system (language) with many concepts having no direct equivalent in the Japanese lexicon. Their definitions are reduced to straight translations that are rote memorised, having the form of occupational therapy in the West but lacking meaning and the power to inform and guide a meaningful, valued practice.

In the spring of 1999, the author was asked to give a two-day workshop on occupational therapy theory to practitioners, educators and students of occupational therapy located in Okayama Prefecture in Western Japan. The plan was straightforward in the workshop leader's mind: take what even North American students find difficult about studying occupational therapy theory and teach it methodically in simplified language over a longer period of time. 'Just slow it all down and use simple language to get the material across and anybody can understand this material'. But it wasn't necessarily a problem of translation, it was the fact that the concepts and principles contained in the foreign theoretical material could not be anchored to or related to meaningfully by these Japanese participants and their common spheres of experience and meaning.

The author had just arrived back to his native Japan from Canada to teach at one of Japan's new baccalaureate occupational therapy programmes, and had not yet made an adequate cultural transition to Japanese social contexts and ways of knowing. The profound differences in world views and divergent spheres of experience that transcended issues of language had not yet been fully comprehended. To add to the challenges, most of the terms found in these transplanted models had no equivalents in the Japanese lexicon. Occupation, for example, with all of the contextual meanings Western occupational therapists had ascribed to it, had been translated as 'sagyou', roughly meaning 'tedious, laborious work' in a Western context. And what do the terms 'personal causation' and 'self-efficacy', which are given meaning in a context of egalitarian social structure, mean in an alternate context structured along principles of hierarchy and collectivism? What is 'leisure' when comprehended from a different orientation to the meaning of productivity in a group-oriented Japanese social context?

After the weekend workshop, participants were reporting that they still could not understand the meaning of occupation nor the other concepts embodied in these North American models. It would be known later that this workshop was yet another workshop of many that the participants had attended in their sincere quest to study and understand occupational therapy theory. Several of the participants would later approach the author for extra study sessions in their attempt to understand *occupational therapy* better. It is significant to note that through a hierarchical social view of phenomena, the problem of not being able to understand theory is usually viewed as a problem of the subordinate than any inadequacy residing in the teacher or in the material being presented. These therapists responded to their inability to grasp imported theory in the following ways: 'I need to study more'; 'I am lacking in intelligence and therefore cannot understand this theory'; 'Americans use MOHO so therefore I should be able to use it too'.

This pattern of inability to comprehend contemporary occupational therapy theory was not limited to this workshop, but was found to be pervasive across the entire nation. Teachers at the various occupational therapy training programmes across Japan will attest to the fact that the same issues and responses to understanding theory exist across the occupational therapy landscape in Japan. The author suspects this to be the case not just in Japan but wherever occupational therapy and the culture it subsumes makes its way into non-mainstream Western communities and avenues of occupational therapy service.

If students and practitioners were still unable to, despite buying all of the prescribed books and attending courses and expensive workshops on OT

Raising a New, Culturally Relevant Conceptual Model of Occupational Therapy from Practice

theory, grasp the theoretical material nor apply it in their practice, what would it take for clients and patients, who have never taken a theory course in occupational therapy, to understand, find meaningful and experience benefit from occupational therapy? Not only had many clinicians given up on trying to understand, let alone explain the bases to their practice to clients, they had also given up on trying to explain their mandate and role to other health care team members.

Occupational therapists were finding their own ways for coping with OT theory and processes so out of sync with their own views and comprehension of reality. Clinicians were saddled with incomprehensible occupational therapy theories and knowledge. They reported experiencing: narrow scope of practice governed by the medical model; unclear professional role and identity; lack of confidence in service delivery; poor understanding of the value of theory and its link to practice; widening gap between academia and the clinical world; and diminishing hope for a more meaningful practice[16].

The effect on professional morale was devastating. Occupational therapists were disempowered from truly enabling their clients in meaningful ways while being denied a vision for the profession and their places within it. They were being defined by the recipe-oriented service delivery forms and techniques which were void of tangible connections to meaning in Japanese daily life. The Canadian Model of Occupational Performance[17] and the Model of Human Occupation[18] were being employed haphazardly as if the esoteric language and inner principles of the models were some kind of code bestowed from heaven that only the most enlightened gurus of occupational therapy could decipher.

Having no tangible narratives or models that held meaning within their own cultural understandings, Japanese therapists were reporting a certain degree of frustration regarding the lack of philosophical and ideological guidelines that defined occupational therapy in a comprehensible way. Their identities as occupational therapists were being jeopardised as they lacked meaningful theory that would aid them in explaining the scope and boundaries of their practice. When the more profound reasons of the theoretical crises befalling Japanese occupational therapy were recognised by the author, he approached a group of concerned occupational therapy practitioners in Okayama prefecture and suggested what seemed audacious at the time. 'Why don't you develop your own model of occupational therapy? If equivalent concepts and principles that could safely describe, explain, guide and predict outcomes in your practice are non-existent, why don't you develop your own, from your own spheres of shared experiences around the meaning of Japanese agency?' The notion was that all of these experienced occupational therapists actually had been attempting to take these imported rehabilitation mandates and reconcile them into their own contexts of practice. Occupational therapy had existed for over 35 years in Japan, so surely there should be something there under the forms of practice that were observable on the surface. To develop a culturally relevant model of occupational therapy, there would need to be ways to uncover or emerge out of real practice contexts, a new set of concepts and principles to represent a working template for a unique and meaningful practice of occupational therapy. This might also entail reconceptualising occupation to mean something in the local cultural context of meanings.

While it may be important to study theories and approaches developed in other nations, what was urgently needed in Japan, as well as other settings, were culturally relevant theories and approaches that were understandable and held meaning for occupational therapists and the societies they belonged to and served. Theories, assessments and approaches that have originated in the local culture or have been adapted by occupational therapists for local use are ultimately needed appropriately to describe, explain and guide meaningful and effective health care for Japanese occupational therapists, students and their society.

In a bold attempt to discover and claim a basic framework for the purpose of describing, explaining and guiding their professional interventions in a culturally appropriate manner, a group of occupational therapists, educators and students in Western Japan embarked on a naturalistic research project that combined heuristic research and grounded theory methodology. Unlike traditional quantitative research that has largely been used to test theory, the research group chose qualitative research approaches to mine original concepts germane to their experience and interpretation of Japanese occupational therapy. Shared experiences, meanings and interpretations of 'health' and 'disability' were also explored. And since the resulting conceptual model was to be derived from Japanese subjects, in Japanese language, using Japanese concepts and metaphors having high contextual meaning, it is suggested that the emerged model represents a culturally relevant theoretical work and one of the first of its kind in Asia.

The core members of this research group initially approached the author to form such a focus group after he had run a sequence of theory workshops for the prefectural occupational therapy association in Western Japan. In particular, a workshop on clinical applications of the Model of Human Occupation, which raised issues of the difficulties appeared to galvanise these clinicians to do *something* to bring more *meaning* into their practice of occupational therapy. These clinicians reported an epiphany regarding why substantial problems applying imported conceptual models were experienced despite much effort and time applied to learning them. Senior members of the group concurred that the epiphany was like a wall of ignorance being cracked, allowing in fresh rays of awareness and enlightenment. At the time, several of the group members expressed having experienced an 'identity crisis' – not knowing what the purpose and meaning of their roles as occupational therapists were to both the context of Japanese healthcare and the society at large. Through those workshops, some came to realise that an absence of culturally relevant and meaningful theory and its relation to practice was apparent and needed to be addressed.

Once the purpose of the focus group – to emerge a culturally relevant explanation of Japanese occupational therapy – was known, participants voluntarily attended monthly sessions. Some participants travelled considerable distances, coming from neighbouring prefectures in order to attend. Thus the inclusion criteria for these sessions were only that the participant had an interest in occupational therapy theory and desired to participate in making their clinical practice theoretically clearer.

Focus Group

The shared experiences of occupational therapists in the Japanese clinical context were mined to emerge concepts, constructs and the relationships between them. The data were analysed to form a structural 'map' of the experience of the practice of occupational therapy in Japan. Grounded Theory, a qualitative research method established by sociologists Glaser and Strauss[19], was initially chosen but the group would eventually come to realise that even research methods were culturally bound and based on certain epistemological perspectives and world views. Two methodological challenges were immediately apparent: focus group dynamics in the tradition of Western qualitative research methods were based on a positivistic assumption that a theory lay hidden in phenomena ready to be emerged; and data collection was dependent on verbal, rational expressions which were prone to the culturally variant rules governing communication. In hierarchically stratified groups, for example, free expression of perspectives can be constrained by seniority of group members as well as the cultural currency that each member brings to the focus group.

Nevertheless, the group proceeded with this qualitative method which involved developing codes, categories and themes inductively rather than imposing predetermined classifications on the data[20]. As the codes and themes surfaced, certain working hypotheses and assertions were drawn from the data.

Participants

The initial sample group was comprised of 20 occupational therapy clinicians ($n = 15$), educators ($n = 3$) and students ($n = 2$), interested in 'theory', organised in a focus group. Mean age was 31.5 years, ranging from 21 to 56 years (SD 9.79). The mean clinical experience in years was 7.3 (range = 13, SD = 3.93). Areas of specialty were varied including physical medicine ($n = 5$), geriatrics (v = 5), mental health ($n = 4$), paediatrics ($n = 3$) and education ($n = 3$). The group met monthly at a central location in the city of Kurashiki, Okayama prefecture, for durations of approximately 6 hours per session (Figure 6.1). The opportunity to talk about concerns about their practice coupled with the hope of being able to do something to develop and improve their occupational therapy seemed to galvanise their interests and commitment to the profession. It would gradually become common to participate in meetings that typically commenced at 7 p.m. and extend on into the following morning. At this point in the research, the author knew that there was a potential for something significant and substantial that these Japanese occupational therapists would be able to give to their compatriots located within Japan and beyond its national borders.

Emerging a Japanese Occupational Therapy Framework

The preliminary sessions were spent reviewing and discussing ideas and issues regarding theory and practice. These sessions were both instructive as well as discursive, serving as a forum to sample participants' ideas as well as expectations of a focus group on Japanese occupational therapy theory. Western cultural practices and norms for rational thought and the place that theory commands in the Western scientific tradition, as well as Japanese ways of perceiving theory, were explored.

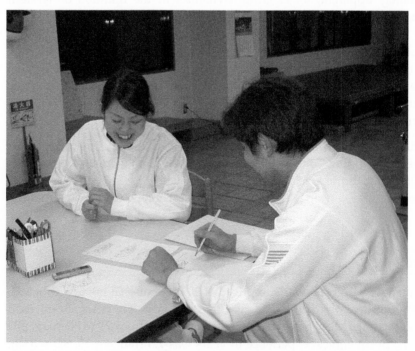

Figure 6.1 The Kawa model was raised out of Japanese occupational therapy practice contexts by clinicians, meeting regularly to discuss their practice issues in cultural context.

It became apparent that the research design needed altering to account for certain cultural and social factors. Though grounded theory and other qualitative research designs appear to be more culturally safe, owing to the freedom this research genre offers for the uncovering of meanings people attach to their experiences, there are certain threats to the reliability of the collected data owing to aspects of the Japanese social. The systematic structure of research is very much an extension of the rational, material and analytical world views shared by many who have been socialised in the West. For one, the social context of egalitarianism and 'equal rights' sanctions the expressions of one's own feelings and thoughts and valuing of others' comments. Westerners in a group may not necessarily temper their verbal participation according to their relations with others set on an age gradient and also may not index their social status and behaviour on the horizontal plane demarking a line between inside (*uchi*) and outside (*soto*) (see Chapter 5). These Japanese institutions of behaviour, social interaction and interpretation of self and reality to some extent can impede or at least influence the quality of data that are drawn from this type of focus group research. In Japanese groups, incumbents are conditioned to speak in turn and it is common for younger, less experienced members to defer to their senior members rather than express themselves freely. Furthermore, in the instance where participants are complete strangers and have no conceivable role or place in the group, they may withdraw their participation completely, void of power, as if they did not exist.

Though grounded theory is widely used in Japan, there are several such methodological areas that warrant change to facilitate adequate harvesting of quality data. Thus, conventional grounded theory, which traditionally relies heavily on interviews and verbally conveyed data, required changes to ensure better quality data from a Japanese population and cultural setting.

In an attempt to overcome these initial threats to the reliability of the forthcoming data, several strategies were employed. The first was to make the purpose of this research known clearly to each group member. It would be necessary for the senior members to allow and even encourage the participation of their junior members. Though virtually impossible to eradicate completely such a hindrance, having all participants aware of the limitations imposed on the data emergence by this social pattern was necessary.

The second measure taken was to structure the data collection to occur in smaller sub-focus groups, in order to decrease any barriers that speaking in front of a larger group might impose. Once again, the same social structures that were expected to influence participation could not be fully controlled, but this was seen to be one more means to minimise the barriers to data emergence. Care was taken to allow therapists to be in groups with others of the same specialty (i.e. psychiatry, geriatrics, paediatrics, etc.). The rationale for this being that the emerged themes and codes would be shared in similar contexts of clinical experiences and meanings.

The third and perhaps most significant measure taken to facilitate the best return of comments and participation was the flexibility given to the sampling method for collecting data. Given the limitations of verbal expression of one's thoughts in the social context, other media such as writing responses on cards or collectively emerging drawn diagrams on pieces of paper or the white board were initially given leeway. Participation and the expression of one's thoughts on an issue were made the foremost task, allowing the researcher freedom to explore different avenues for emerging data and subsequent codes. As elaborated in the preamble, the notion that the participants might regard and value phenomena in 'situational' or 'socially relativistic ways' could not be dismissed. When asking a question such as: 'how is disability regarded in your clinical setting?', the respondent may express having considerable difficulty understanding the enquiry and exactly in what context to place the issue of disability. Given the flexible nature of Japanese person's interpretations of reality based on situation and 'ba', and the primacy given to the social over self, the boundaries of the social context in question may need to be set before one's opinion is assembled and expressed.

Data Sources

Prior to the first formal set of group gatherings, intensive, focused interviews were conducted with four of the core members of the research participants. These interviews yielded the general rationale and boundaries of the ensuing research. The main outcomes of these sessions were the unanimous discontent and discouragement that these therapists had felt about the current state of their practices. There were concerns about the dubious *meaning* of occupational therapy. These therapists expressed concerns about the vagueness of occupational therapy's purpose. The purported aim of occupational therapy intervention was difficult to reconcile with their learned ideas about health care, and they were unsure whether occupational therapy really made a difference to the health outcomes of their clients. Three of the four expressed an imminent 'identity crisis', stating that Japanese occupational therapists knew very little theory – at least theory that made sense to them, to guide and explain their practices. And having worked within the Japanese health care institutions, they expressed dissatisfaction with the apparent biomedical perspective of occupational therapy. They also unanimously expressed an interest in *theory* and felt that if it were possible, a (culturally) meaningful frame of reference for Japanese occupational therapists was needed.

Going into the formal sessions, two initial open questions were put to the group: 'How do you as Japanese occupational therapists conceive of the concepts of health and disability and illness?' and 'What, if there is any, role or relation does occupational therapy have with these concepts?' The rationale for these questions were founded in the understanding that if Western occupational therapy theory linked occupation, or doing, to what was deemed essential to Western people's experiences of well-being, a new culturally relevant model should attempt to explore a new definition of occupation that would link the concept to something that the local population deemed essential to their perspectives and experiences of well-being. At this point, the author had taken a participant-observer role to help facilitate the exchange of the participants' ideas. Participants were encouraged by the author to think about the concepts during the weeks between gatherings. It began to dawn on the group members that this was not going to be a 'benkyou-kai' (literally translated into 'study-group') as encountered in other 'research group' experiences, where learning processes typically follow a hierarchical top-down dynamic, but that each and everyone's experiences and takes on reality would count towards some type of important process. Responses were recorded graphically on white boards and discussed interactively in small groups and then with the larger whole. Notes and video footage were taken to record the conversations as well as to record thoughts from a cross-cultural perspective.

This initial phase provided a general backdrop onto which occupational therapy could be reflected. The primary research question was then raised: *'What is the meaning of Japanese occupational therapy?'* To focus the enquiry further, the alternate questions: *'What is your role in Japanese society?'*; *'What do you do and why?'*; *'Who are your clients and what are you concerned with?'* were used. Inductively, it was believed that ideas about the social construction of occupational therapy, disability and health, in Japan would naturally emerge from the data.

As mentioned earlier, conventional grounded theory methods may encounter difficulties in light of the Japanese strong situational regard of realities and preferred methods of expressing and communicating their inner held thoughts. One other adjunct to the grounded theory process was the use of file cards in a procedure of brain-storming in which the subject could convey their thoughts in written, rather than verbal form. The advantage to this procedural approach appears to be at least threefold. The first advantage being that the subject is able to defer others' scrutiny over one's comments to a later time. The second is the dimension of time afforded to participants as they gather their thoughts rather than having to express themselves in an instance. The assembled comments can be viewed vis-à-vis other comments in 'real-time', immediately allowing comparison of comments. In other words, participants need not be held back from sharing their thoughts due to rules of speaking in turn according to hierarchical status in Japanese social situations. The rationale for allowing these variations to conventional data collection in grounded theory is in keeping with the research objective and looking for the best possible ways to emerge data in light of known cultural and social factors.

The use of file-cards in the data collection process was reportedly reminiscent for some of the participants, particularly those working in mental health, of a brainstorming method locally known as 'KJ Houritsu'[21], or translated – the KJ method. In this method, cards or slips of paper are apparently used, arranged on conditions of similarity or adherence to particular themes, and pasted onto a large piece of paper, to form a graphic representation of a particular subject matter. This method is reportedly popular in group activities in Japanese mental health programmes and settings. A variation of this method was used in this research as its familiarity was seen to be conducive in emerging quality data.

In total, the group met over 50 times over a 2.5 year period. The amount of time taken to emerge the subsequent initial model was estimated to be approximately 250 hours. Prompt and thorough recording of data was taken seriously to ensure rigour in the methodology. All notes were logged and photographs taken of the sorted and assembled data. This included the initial, secondary and tertiary data collection stages, as well as follow-up interactions. Some of the sessions were videotaped, yielding just over 6 hours of graphic data (Figure 6.2). All data were recorded in writing and initially transcribed and coded in SSPS 10.01. The database was then transferred to Microsoft Excel to make file sharing easier among participants.

Data Collection and Analysis

The main analysis consisted of the usual requirements that characterise conventional grounded theory methodology. The process of emerging a conceptual model requires examining each datum and analysing it through repeated sortings, codings and comparisons. The data were emerged from the general enquiry; *'What is the meaning of Japanese occupational therapy?'* Other questions were added to clarify the question for those who needed more

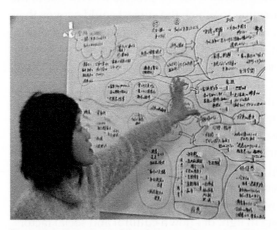

Figure 6.2 Early photo of the data recording and analyses process. Visual recording and analyses of data were common in the research process. All processes were videotaped (this image was reduced from vtr footage taken in 1999).

structure to complete the task. These included: *'What is your role in Japanese society?'*; *'What do you do (in regard to intervention) and why?*; *'Who are your clients?'*; *'What are you concerned with in your work?'*; *'How do you (Japanese OTs) define and regard "health", "disability"?'*

Recorded data from interviews, brainstorming sessions and videotape were put through the process known as 'open coding'[22]. Here minute sections of text constructed from singular words, phrases and sentences are gathered according to the guiding research questions. Strauss and Corbin state that the process of open coding 'fractures the data and allows one to identify some categories, their properties and dimensional locations' (p. 97). In the process, the participants' language (both Japanese and professional jargon) was used to guide the development of code and category labels. The English translations are used here for the purpose of reporting. The open coding phase yielded 398 responses, which were coded and placed into the data pool. These codes and emergent categories were systematically compared and contrasted, emerging even more complex and inclusive categories.

This initial process of open coding was followed by another step in the methodology, which Strauss and Corbin refer to as 'Axial Coding'[22]. In this phase, the raised codes are critically examined through a rigorous process of comparing and contrasting, with an eye towards forming groups of common or connected data. One by one, each raised code was looked at with the intended meaning confirmed by the parties that donated the code. It is important to note here that in the confirmation process, each code had to be explained in terms of its situational circumstance, as if the concept or code could not be understood unless the circumstance surrounding the code was clearly described. This was remarkable in the author's point of view, affirming the Japanese world view of flexible truths – truths that are situated and defined in concert with context (rather than being reflected to some universal norm or standard). Situational relativism was apparent throughout the procedure and highlighted the importance that context or 'ba' plays as an important factor in the interpretation and judgement of realities for these Japanese therapists.

One other observation made by the researcher at this point of the analysis was how most problems or concepts raised in these codes were tied to a social reference to some capacity, rather than to some other concept like 'agency', which is reflexive to a significant extent.

Many of these codes during the axial coding process were 'tagged' with 3M 'sticky notes' on which a brief description could be written. Later as these codes were segregated into groupings, colour coded tags were utilised to organise the data. Groupings of data along certain themes began to emerge and tentative categories were formed (Figure 6.3). These tentative categories were:

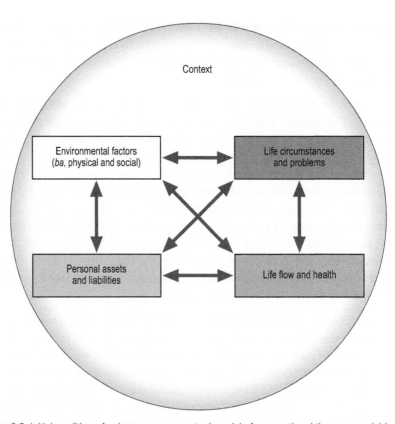

Figure 6.3 Initial rendition of a Japanese conceptual model of occupational therapy, as yielded by a modified grounded theory approach.

- Life flow and health
- Environmental factors (social, 'ba', physical barriers)
- Life circumstances and problems
- Personal assets and liabilities
- Occupational therapy intervention.

Selective coding, which symbolises the process of selecting a 'central concept' of concern and 'systematically relating it to the other categories, validating those relationships (by searching for confirming and disconfirming examples), and filling in categories that need(ed) further refinement and development'[22] (p. 116).

Perhaps as important as the concepts/categories that emerged from the data was the structure of the principles relating these concepts together. Whereas most rational models show some direction in the relation between concepts, relationships among these emerged concepts were conspicuous by the complete absence of linearity and direction. Each of the concepts was tied to each and all of the other concepts, with double-headed arrows. This structure inferred that no single concept held a central, primary position nor did any one single concept hold greater value or emphasis over any of the others. This configuration and structure could be described as a dynamic rubric in which any disruption or change in magnitude and quality of any one concept would affect the magnitude and quality of all of the other concepts. None of the concepts were considered solitary and distinctly separate from the others. All elements of self, other, circumstance and environment were integrated and inseparable – conjuring images of the East Asian cosmological myth presented in earlier chapters of this book. One non-Japanese occupational therapist who looked at this result commented with incredulity: 'this is like an amoeba – you simply cannot liken the human system and its relationship to occupation to an amoeba!' Another reaction to this preliminary model, from a Western cultural perspective was: 'where is the self in all of this – I can't see where the person is here'.

Although the core guiding question was: 'what is the meaning of occupational therapy?', it was interesting to discover the participants' preference and emphasis on the category or concept of 'life' and 'life force'. There was a shared need to anchor these emerged topics, including 'occupational therapy' to something essential to Japanese perspectives of 'being'. Previously encountered foreign conceptual models placed the concept of 'occupation', with emphases on 'self' and 'doing' and deemed by Western occupational therapists as essential to life, at its core.

Emergence of the River Metaphor

Prior to the final stage of analysis, which is the 'selective coding' phase according to Strauss and Corbin's nomenclature, various members of the project conjured up several drawings to summarise the interrelationships between the emerged categories. One member proclaimed that the Japanese person's life, social circumstances and the purpose of occupational therapy could be explained by the metaphor of a river, or 'kawa' in Japanese. Up to this point in the research project, the Japanese therapists were complying with the author's directions to produce a model made up of boxes and arrows in the usual logical, linear configuration. While the author was initially content to see a linear model emerge, the Japanese therapists raised a resounding cry of agreement when the suggestion was forwarded that the model could be better explained by an image of nature – the river. The Japanese person's life being depicted by a metaphor of nature seemed like a natural interpretation for a society whose cosmologies are based on a naturalistic paradigm and whose ideations of humans are constructively inseparable from nature, society and deities. Most important was the unanimous consent given for the emerged conceptual model to take on this metaphorical shape. It will be argued that over conventional linear diagrams to depict models that describe some aspect of the human (social) experience, a three-dimensional image of a familiar metaphor such as a river, is legitimised on the merit of its interpretation, meaning and profound explanatory power, to the population from which the model was emerged, and for which the model is intended (Figure 6.4).

The existing categories were renamed by the research participants to fit the metaphor of the river as follows:

1 Life and health was ascribed the concept of 'water' or *mizu* in Japanese. A person's life was depicted to be a fluid transition over life circumstances (represented in the river metaphor as rocks or *iwa*). The volume of water flowing (unimpeded by rocks and debris) was a symbol for 'life flow'. Greater water volume would symbolise a better, 'fuller' state of health and well-being. The fluid constitution of water was also congruent with a less clearly defined construction of 'self'.

2 Life circumstances and problems were assigned the metaphor of 'rocks' or *iwa* in Japanese. They exist in all sizes and are seen mostly as a negative influence on the flow of water (life). They can form or appear suddenly and ominously in the water, just like illnesses, injuries, challenges and difficulties occur in life, or they could have existed from early in life, such as with congenital conditions. It is their size and compounding effect, when congregated with other rocks and material that can affect the volume of water that flows at a given point of the river. They are either directly or indirectly seen to have a relation to the social environment depicting the social consequences of what might be medically described as physical or mental insults. They form ominous relations with the river's sides and bottom collaboratively to impede life-water flow.

3 Personal assets and liabilities were referred to as 'driftwood' or *ryuboku*. These represent incidental factors that can affect a person's problem

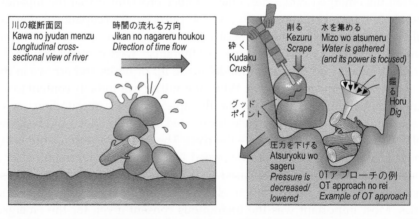

Figure 6.4 Early drawings (reduced to two-colour from colour) recording the transformation of the initial linear model (see Figure 6.3) to the metaphorical presentation of life depicted by a river. The longitudinal view (left) shows the temporal quality of the metaphor. The cross-section (right) carries all of the main concepts of the model and their possible interactions, or principles. Drawings by Terumi Hatsutori and Mayumi Okuda; used with permission.

positively or negatively, given a difficult circumstance or challenge. Driftwood can drift in to spaces between the rocks and between the rocks and river sides/bottom to block water flow. They could also potentially drift into problematic areas, to move other impeding structures away to enlarge the flow or enable a new channel for the water to flow through.

4 Environmental factors (social, *ba*, physical barriers) were ascribed the term *torimaki* in Japanese or the bottom (*kawa zoko*) and sides (*kawa no soku heki*) of the river which contain the flow of water (life). It is mainly made up of social factors and *ningen-kankei* or 'human relations'. Immediate family, friends or any other party who has penetrated through the *tanin* (stranger) barrier to gain a significant level of intimacy with the core person.

5 Strategic points for occupational therapy interventions were typified by weak areas of the structure of the blocking elements and/or spaces between these elements that could be exploited ultimately to allow greater water flow. Occupational Therapy Intervention was seen to be represented by the service of sending or directing 'water' over small openings or weak points between rocks or between rocks and the river walls and floor. Occupational therapy is thus conceptualised as a force or intervention that seeks to strengthen or increase water flow by looking for every opportunity to assist the client to overcome life-flow barriers and other challenges. If at all possible, it is the patient's own power or any other exploitable power source, such as elements of the physical and social environments, that is used in the process of increasing the size of the waterway. Thus, a wider role for occupational therapy, to intervene in the environmental realm is also possible.

The above stated five categories were taken into the selective coding phase, where each code in each category was rigorously scrutinised yet again. These were sorted again, compared and contrasted until the categories were saturated. By saturation, we mean that all of the codes emerged from the previous phases could be reconciled in one of the five core categories and that no new codes or categories were emerged. For the criteria used to determine the 'core' condition of a given category, we defer to Strauss[23]. The criteria were: (a) a category's centrality in relation to other categories; (b) frequency of a category's occurrence in the data; (c) its inclusiveness and the ease with which it related to other categories; (d) clarity of its implications for a more general theory; (e) its movement towards theoretical power as details of a category were worked out; and (f) its allowance for maximum variation in terms of dimensions, properties, conditions, consequences and strategies.

Results

The conceptual model depicting Japanese occupational therapy, evolved from a modified grounded theory approach based on Strauss and Corbin's framework[22] is presented in Figure 6.5. It is purposefully presented in the

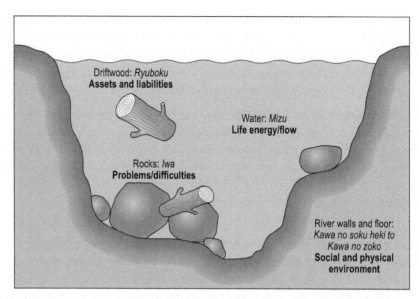

Figure 6.5 Cross-section view of the early Kawa model showing the basic concepts in Japanese and in English.

metaphorical form, rather than a static two-dimensional linear diagram, such as Figure 6.3, to capture certain fluid elements of the Japanese occupational therapists' explanations of their shared experiences and meanings. There are certain remarkable aspects of the emerged model that warrant special attention. These aspects pertaining to the social construction of Japanese occupational therapy are offered here.

The Context of Japanese Occupational Therapy

The social context in which occupational therapy finds its purpose and meaning was emerged from the clinical situational experiences shared by the occupational therapists in the group. The context is based on the Japanese occupational therapy client, whose humanesque figure cannot be seen so clearly in the metaphorical illustration of the model. The 'self', which is usually placed at the centre of Western depictions of the social, is arguably a trait of a specific world view that values such ideals as *individualism* and *self-determinism*.

This is a depiction that makes allowances for a non-universal, particularistic view of human experience and meaning, in which situational ethic, and situation-influenced interpretations of truth are permitted and validated. Universal assumptions about the singular goal of independence (as opposed to interdependence), personal achievement and self-actualisation, which are common in the West, are placed aside. In fact, this appears to be a depiction of Japanese social experience that includes various elements and aspects of society and nature inside, and an inseparable part, of the definition of the self.

The main concept of this emerged model is *mizu* (water). Mizu symbolises 'life' and the will or drive to live. It is one aspect of the central human that touches every other component of 'reality'. It is synonymous with 'health'. When one is living life to its fullest, a state of contentment and satisfaction, the river metaphor is depicted as a 'full' river in which the volume of water flowing is large. Problems that warrant the intervention of an occupational therapist occur when, due to life circumstances, (rocks – *iwa*), environmental factors (social and physical environs – *torimaki*), or some aspect within or related to the individual themselves (driftwood – *ryuboku*), the flow of life is impeded (see Figure 6.5). The essence of occupational therapy is to assist in making one's life flow stronger and more voluminous – no matter what the age, gender or level of capacity of the client might be.

The environment or *torimaki*, which is mainly interpreted in the social circumstance, forms arguably the most important concept next to 'life' itself. The sides and floor of the river bound and give ultimate shape to the water flowing within it. It serves as the one singular point of reference from which all things and phenomena can be judged. The shape of the *torimaki* (social network, family, etc.) can assist the flow or act against it. When it projects into the stream, which symbolises a problematic social environment, it can catch other elements that come down the watercourse as well as butting up against a rock, transforming simple problems into more complex, stubborn types. Occupational therapy was constructed in a way in which the therapist will develop a keen eye to look opportunistically for thin spaces between the physical elements in the client's river. If there are no spaces to exploit, the occupational therapist may need to go beyond merely directing (the therapeutic activity of the patient) and find a particular weak spot to make a way for the life flow to get through. *Seken*[24] (significant social 'others') and various other aspects of the Japanese social cannot be overlooked. In a collectivist society, where belonging is *everything*, one's interface with the social becomes more important than any egocentric, individual, reference such as self-efficacy and personal causation.

Rocks or *iwa* symbolise circumstantial problems, usually within one's own body, or can combine with some of the other elements to compound a problem. *Iwa* come in all different types, shapes and sizes. The most frequent being a physical impairment or complaint, but inevitably, it is its abutment with the social element (*torimaki*) that emerges its reliable forms and meanings. For a collectively oriented person, how the surrounding social interprets one's own physical or mental impairment appears to have significant bearing on how large the problem is perceived to be, as well as the best way to treat it. Problems with social ramifications often require socially-oriented intervention strategies. The occupational therapist may elect to assist the client to increase their capabilities, thus effectively making the size of the problem more manageable.

Driftwood or *ryuboku* symbolises personal assets and liabilities. These represent incidental factors that can affect a person's problem positively or negatively, given a difficult circumstance or challenge. These should by no means be construed as personal traits or attributes only. Driftwood can lodge between rocks or between the sides of the river and a rock to compound existing difficulties. On the other hand, a piece of driftwood might come along and dislodge some structure to make a way to increase flow. These are elements that can also mimic those elements of good or bad fortune that come into play at the time of the person's illness and subsequent need for occupational therapy intervention. This can come in the form of material elements such as a wealth or lack of resources and money or immaterial such as a particular value patterns or character traits that can have an effect on one's performance in an active therapeutic programme. It can also refer to extraordinary social relationships with powerful individuals or groups in the community – a factor that cannot be underestimated in Japanese society.

The occupational therapist may desire to evaluate the client holistically and consider all of these peripheral elements in order to understand the client's situation. Intervention may involve minimising the effects of these liabilities, as well as utilising the client's assets towards progress in rehabilitation. These outcomes and the emerged conceptual model have been tested in various clinical settings as a test of face and construct validity. In the previous four

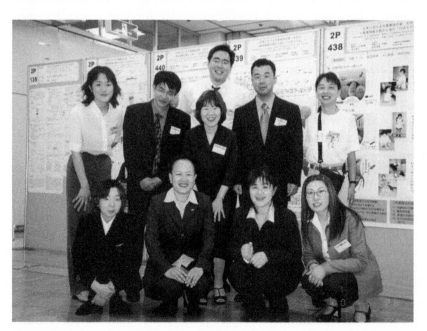

Figure 6.6 Ten of the original members, all clinicians, who participated in developing the Kawa model pose for a group photograph following their presentations of six landmark papers on a new model of occupational therapy at the 34th National Congress of the Japanese Association of Occupational Therapy, May 26, 2000, Yokohama, Japan.

years where clinicians in various parts of Japan have tested the model, the preliminary results have been, on the whole, very encouraging.

REFERENCES

[1] Iwama M. The issue is ... toward culturally relevant epistemologies in occupational therapy. American Journal of Occupational Therapy 2003; 57(5):582–588

[2] Gans H. Middle American Individualism. New York: The Free Press; 1988

[3] Kerlinger FN. Foundations of Behavioural Research. New York: Holt, Rinehart & Winston; 1973

[4] Bellah R. Beyond Belief: Essays on Religion in a Post Traditional World. New York: Harper & Row; 1991

[5] Berque A. Identification of the self in relation to the environment. In: Rosenberger N (ed). Japanese Sense of Self. Cambridge: Cambridge University Press; 1992; 93–104

[6] Lebra TS. Japanese Patterns of Behavior. Honolulu: University of Hawaii Press; 1976

[7] Bandura A. Self-Efficacy: Toward a Unifying Theory of Behavioral Change. Psychological Review 1977; (84):191–215

[8] deCharms R. Personal Causation: The Internal Affective Determinants of Behavior. New York: Academic Press; 1968

[9] Watanabe S. The Peasant Soul of Japan. New York: St Martin's; 1980

[10] Nakane C. Tate shakai no ningen kankei [Human Relations in a Vertical Society]. Tokyo: Kodansha; 1970

[11] Doi T. The Anatomy of Self: The Individual Versus Society. Tokyo: Kodansha International; 1985

[12] Doi T. Amae no kozo [The Anatomy of Dependence]. Tokyo: Kobundo;1971 (in Japanese)

[13] Kielhofner G. A model of human occupation. Part 3: Benign and vicious cycles. American Journal of Occupational Therapy 1980; 34:731–737

[14] Kielhofner G, Burke JP. A model of human occupation. Part 1: Conceptual framework and content. American Journal of Occupational Therapy 1980; 34:572–581

[15] Miller R. What is theory and why does it matter? In: Miller R, Sieg K, Ludwig F, Shortridge S, Van Deusen J (eds), Six Perspectives on Theory for the Practice of Occupational Therapy. Rockville, Aspen Publishers Inc; 1988

[16] Iwama M. A social perspective on the construction of occupational therapy in Japan. Unpublished doctoral dissertation. Takahashi: Kibi International University; 2001

17 Canadian Association of Occupational Therapists. Enabling Occupation: an Occupational Therapy Perspective. Toronto: CAOT Publications; 1997

18 Kielhofner G. A Model of Human Occupation: Theory and Application, 2nd edn. Baltimore: Williams and Wilkins; 1995

19 Glaser B, Strauss A. The Discovery of Grounded Theory. Chicago: Aldine; 1967

20 Glaser BG. Theoretical Sensitivity. Mill Valley: Sociology Press; 1978

21 Kawakita J. Hassou hou; souzou sei kaihatsu no tame ni. Tokyo: Chuo Kouronsha; 1967

22 Strauss A, Corbin J. Basics of Qualitative Research: Grounded Theory Procedures and Techniques. Newbury Park: Sage; 1990

23 Strauss A. Qualitative Analysis for Social Scientists. New York: Cambridge University Press; 1987

24 Kuwayama T. The reference other orientation. In: Rosenberger N (ed.), Japanese Sense of Self. Cambridge: Cambridge University Press; 1992; 121–151

An Overview of the Kawa Model

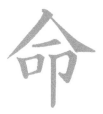

命

The philosophical and ontological bases underlying the Kawa model are originally located in Japanese social and cultural contexts. The social and cultural conditions and circumstances from which a model's concepts and their interrelations have been drawn need to be fully understood and appreciated in order to grasp fully the model's potential and appropriate application. The Kawa model attempts to explain occupational therapy's overall purpose, strategies for interpreting a client's circumstances and clarify the rationale and application of occupational therapy within the client's particular social and cultural context. Though occupational therapists will and have already adapted the model to their own particular social and cultural contexts, readers of this chapter will see that the description of the model's components in their original form is culturally situated. In keeping with a constructionist perspective on how concepts and other symbolic representations of phenomena are situated in place and time, the inseparable nature of creator and created is purposely laid bare for all to see. While examining the Kawa model's structure and content, readers may want to compare the original Japanese interpretations of the river metaphor with their own constructions and interpretations of the same. By doing so, occupational therapists may discover the often overlooked necessity to examine critically theoretical material in occupational therapy practice. Occupational therapists are encouraged to explore their own rationale for adapting and utilising the Kawa model to their own (cultural) practice contexts.

One can readily see that this original Asian model's structure and content depart significantly from the familiar structure and content of occupational therapy models that were raised and imported from Western cultural contexts. Even before the model took on the metaphor of the river, which holds profound meaning in many cultures, particularly in Japan, elements previously deemed essential in Western explanations of occupational therapy, such as the central incumbency of the individual, and a tacit understanding of humans as occupational beings, or occupation typified as the interface between self and environment, were being critically challenged. Consistent with a cosmology or world view that perceives reality as a single integrated entity (see Figure 3.1), the resultant Kawa model raised by these clinical experts located in Japan took on the form of a circular, relational dynamic. In this dynamic, the four basic factors of environment, life circumstances, personal assets and liabilities, and life flow and health, combine to form a unique configuration set in a particular instance in time and place. The stage has now been set for occupational therapy intervention.

The absence of a central, discrete, physically bounded *self*, substituted by a configuration of several elements which, when combined, make up the *self*, reflects a less rational depiction of human existence typified so strongly in Western narratives on personal agency. The absence of a centrally placed discrete self also renders occupation, in the Western sense of the concept, a different purpose, imbuing it with a quality that is less instrumental and purpose driven. The construal of self is more in line with the 'primitive' cosmological world view in which the self is resigned to being just another (inseparable) element of nature and context. It is interesting to be reminded at this juncture that the Japanese term for self – *jibun* – literally means 'self-part', or 'one's share' (of the whole). Westerners looking at the Kawa model for the first time may be concerned about where the 'self' is located in the model. The self is there but construed in a different way. Instead of self placed in opposition to nature or the surrounding environment, the self in the Kawa model is construed as being an integral part of nature. Instead of the imperative to control nature and circumstance, the alternative view is to yield to nature and circumstance and find ways to live in harmony with them.

All elements in nature, including humans, are profoundly connected. In Western rational views of life there is a tendency to treat elements of nature as discretely separate entities. This tendency coincides with how we make sense of and treat social processes and phenomena like disability, for instance. In the West, the experience of disability is often constructed as a medical issue, contained in the human body and treated more or less as a tragedy of the individual, rather than a collective experience. The Kawa metaphor allows us to see disability from and as a collective experience. When the self is seen as a river, all of the elements including self, society, and circumstances are constructed as elements of one, inseparable whole, where all things are connected and difficult to comprehend in isolation. In this world view, the consequences and impact of a particular disability emanate broadly to a wider social sphere. Ask any person who has had the experience of living with a family member with a disability, they will most likely report that all of their lives have been affected and changed profoundly, and that the experience of disability is a complex and collective one rather than one that is limited and contained within the individual. The Kawa framework forces the occupational therapist to appreciate such phenomena and experiences of well-being in a broader context rather than as something seen in isolation and residing more or less within the person. Like a river, changes to one aspect of the water course, in the river sides and walls, driftwood and rocks, will end up affecting the entire river and its reaches.

Rationally minded observers may regard the relative vagueness (*aimai*) with which the concepts of this model are related as antithetical to the whole notion of theory and rational process. For those who live reality within Japan's collectives, truth and ontology are often viewed to be situational and socially relevant. Such an orientation gives credence to multiple ways of interpreting reality, making the client's viewpoint of his or her predicament the ultimate perspective. Universal definitions and laws for explaining truth and reality are inadequate and rendered impotent in such particular social contexts.

When the Kawa model was being uncovered, traditional linear explanations of phenomena, as exemplified by the original concepts emerged through the grounded theory process, were abandoned for a metaphor that held deeper and clearer meanings for Japanese people. It is important to note that a metaphor of nature, a river in this case, was preferred over a more 'scientific' depiction seen in the initial two-dimensional, 'box and arrow' graphic illustration (see Figure 6.3). The metaphor appeared to have greater and more profound dimensions of meaning than the physically linear constrained box and arrow diagram. The dimensions of what the Western person might refer to as 'affective' and 'spiritual' were better captured by the metaphorical presentation. When pressed to answer why the metaphor of the river was particularly important and preferred over the original box and arrow rendition, one of the Japanese Kawa model research leaders provided the following eloquent rationale:

> The river, historically, has been a very common and important motif in Japanese literature and arts, such as the great hit song by Hibari Misora, 'Like a river flowing'. Great literary works utilising the river metaphor include 'Ho-Jo-Ki' by Choumei Kamono and 'Deep River' by Shuusaku Endo. When we come in touch with such works, annotations such as, 'rivers are metaphors of life', would seem superfluous. However, the river evokes in itself a very rich picture of mental imagery for a Japanese. A projection method developed in Japan called 'fukei kousei hou' also uses the river as 'a metaphor of unconscious flow'. By looking at this holistic picture of our clients and by using such images that flow right deep inside our hearts, we may sympathise with their *komari* (problems) as people who live just like ourselves, otherwise we may understand their *komari* as something that happens to someone else somewhere in life. The clients that we treat and support are living persons. An approach without such sympathy carries the risk of being superficial and an affront to our clients[1].

Shared symbolic meaning of the *kawa* (river) extends deeper to include the sub-concepts that form parts of the metaphor. The use of the symbolic meanings of water, for instance, also raises a constellation of profound meanings for many people. Water is essential for life, it is pure, perpetual and rejuvenating. Water also depicts the course of life itself; originating from the heavens, flowing down mountains and eventually to the sea, to be cycled again into the heavens. Like water, the strategy for rehabilitating is not directly and rationally to confront the perceived problem head on but rather to bend and flex and adapt one's circumstance to the circumstances of the surrounding environment. Taken this way, Japanese occupational therapy intervention may not necessarily focus on unilateral purposeful actions but rather support the client to cope and adapt to a constellation of factors interfacing and constructing that person's problem(s). The focal points for occupational therapy intervention are located wherever the water flow can be increased. The purpose of occupational therapy is not necessarily to increase the individual's self-efficacy, but to examine all relevant parts of nature (context) with the aim to facilitate one's *life flow*. A fundamental premise of the Kawa model is that it is holistic in its views of the client, and that the term 'client' is understood to be as much a collective as it might be an individual.

This culturally relevant model, whether in its initial linear form or in its metaphorical form, provides a set of meaningful symbols that most members of Japanese society (including clients, their families, therapists and health team members) share. The promising and profound explanatory power of this particular metaphor, which was congruent with the initial model raised through this research, is what qualifies it as an appropriate structural map to explain the process of occupational therapy in certain social-cultural contexts.

Structure and Concepts

Reconceptualising Occupation and Occupational Therapy in Cultural Context

Structure of the River As a Metaphor for 'Life Energy' or 'Life Flow'

We begin by introducing the metaphor or image of a river as it occurs in nature as a symbolic representation of life. Instead of life being explained from an existential perspective, in which the self is the focal and ceded the most privileged position of the narrative, self is seen, and treated, in context of all elements in the subject's frame. The view that constructs doing, accomplishment, failure, well-being or disability, for example, as individual embodiment is but an illusion from this perspective. The context is seen to set certain conditions in which a particular action or occupation occurs. The surrounding social and physical environment can, to a significant extent, influence the meaning and value ascribed to an action or phenomenon, as well as contribute to the definitions of what constitutes optimal or undesirable states of being. In this way, the surrounding contexts are given much more credence in determining one's state of being. The surrounding context can enable and disable people.

The complex dynamic that characterises an Eastern perspective of harmony in life between self and context might be best explained through a familiar metaphor[2] of nature. The river is employed as a symbol for the life course. It has its beginning at higher elevations – perhaps in the mountains where clouds drop their heavy loads; where glaciers fed from ice formed aeons ago melt and transform, or underground springs yield their bounty. What may begin as a little rill grows into a stream. Streams can become brooks, which after gathering momentum and greater volume, become creeks. Creeks, like rivers can also combine and split, can flow at different speeds and meander around various structures. Rivers can cease to flow by drying up, by being dammed by natural or man-made actions, by flowing into a terminal lake or into the vast sea. Wherever the river flows, the profound and complex

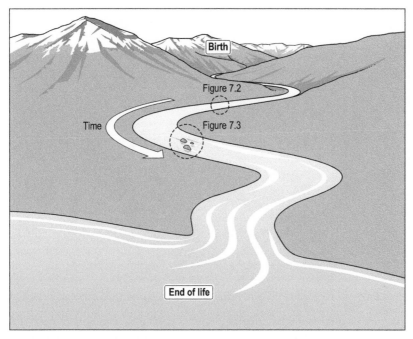

Figure 7.1 Life is like a river, flowing from birth to end of life.

interrelation of other elements of nature become apparent. As other elements of nature participate in the life or flow of a river, so the river also participates in the other. Vital relationships form between all elements in a context/frame and a balance or 'harmony' comes into being. It is a balance that reflects the interrelated nature of the elements quite unlike the artificial, mechanical metaphor of the individual as a 'system' oriented to subdue and exert control over circumstance and an objectified environment.

Life is a complex, profound journey that flows through time and space, *like a river* (Figure 7.1). An optimal state of well-being in one's life or *river*, can be metaphorically portrayed by an image of strong, deep, unimpeded flow. Aspects of the environment and phenomenal circumstances, like certain structures found in a river, can influence and effect that flow. Rocks (life circumstances), walls and bottom (environment), driftwood (assets and liabilities), are all inseparable parts of a river that determine its boundaries, shape and flow (Figure 7.2).

In the prevailing (Western) narratives of occupational therapy, the concept of occupation has been essentially tied to individual health and well-being. Occupation interpreted in this existential, individual-centric way has been problematic to many who do not share these same rational value patterns and world views. When the Western construction of occupation does not exist in many non-English lexicons, there is a need to re-examine the concept of occupation through different cultural lenses – preferably through the cultural

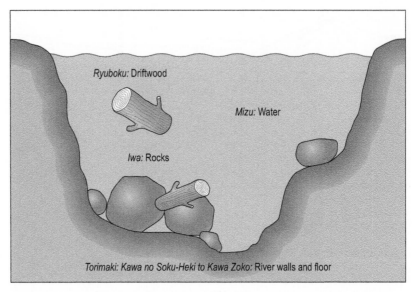

Ryuboku: Driftwood

Mizu: Water

Iwa: Rocks

Torimaki: Kawa no Soku-Heki to Kawa Zoko: River walls and floor

Figure 7.2 Cross-section view of the early Kawa model showing the basic concepts in Japanese and in English.

lenses of the client. For the Japanese originators of the Kawa model, the river is symbolic of life and occupation is reconceptualised to be the flow of water in this river. Without water flowing, there can be no river. Without occupation, in the context of this cosmological view of all elements in a frame or context inextricably connected, there can be no life. In this way, one's own or one's group's occupations are interwoven and connected to the occupation of others. Well-being is a collective phenomenon. Occupational therapy's purpose in this metaphorical representation of human being, then, is to enable and enhance *life flow* – a flow that encompasses self and context.

Mizu (water)

Mizu is Japanese for 'water', and metaphorically represents the subject's *life energy* or *life flow*. Fluid, pure, spirit, filling, cleansing and renewing, are only some of the meanings and functions commonly associated with this natural element. In the model's introduction in various parts of the world removed from Japan, culturally specific interpretations or symbolic meanings of water have been apparent. What are your clients' symbolic understandings of water? The cultural meanings with which one views these concepts will have significant bearing on the utility of this model in one's practice.

Just as people's lives are bounded and shaped by their surroundings, people and circumstances, the water flowing as a river touches the rocks, sides and banks and all other elements that form its context. Water envelops, defines and affects these other elements of the river in a similar way to which the same elements affect the water's volume, shape and flow rate. When life energy or flow weakens, the occupational therapy client, whether defined as individual or collective, can be described as unwell, or in a state of disharmony. When it

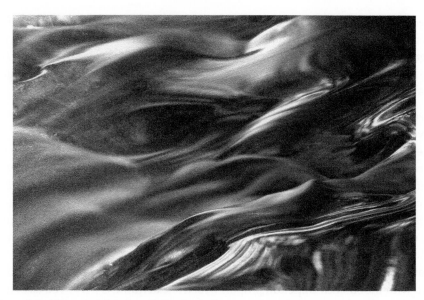

Figure 7.3 Water, what does it symbolise for you?

stops flowing altogether – as when the river releases into a vast ocean – end of life is signified.

In a similar way to which water in its liquid state adopts its form from its container, people in many collective-oriented societies often interpret the social as a shaper of individual selves and groups. Sharing a view of the cosmos that rejects the rational separations of the surrounding world into discrete parts, collectively oriented people tend to place enormous value on the *self* embedded in relationships. There is greater value in 'belonging[3] and 'interdependence[4,5], than in unilateral agency and in individual determinism. In such experience, the interdependent self is deeply influenced and even determined by the surrounding social context, at a given time and place, in a similar way to which water in a river, at any given point, will vary in form, flow direction, rate, volume and clarity. The 'driving force' of one's life is interconnected with others sharing the same social frame or *ba[5]*, in a similar way in which water touches, connects and relates all elements of a river that have varying effect upon its form and flow.

With so much of our consciousness focused on the independent, agent self, there may be a tendency to overlook or de-emphasise the importance that place and context play in determining the form, functions and meanings of people's *doings*. Through the vantage of the Kawa model, a subject's state of well-being coincides with life flow. Occupational therapy's overall purpose in this context is to enhance life flow, regardless of whether it is interpreted at the level of the individual, institution, organisation, community or society. Just as there are constellations of interrelated factors/structures in a river that affect its flow, a rich combination of internal and external circumstances and structures in a client's life context inextricably determine his or her *life flow*. In order for occupational therapists to enable this life flow, it is essential that occupational therapists acquire the knowledge set, experiences and relevant skills defined by the appropriate cultural frame, to understand the multidimensional dynamics of and meanings held in the client's context of daily living.

Torimaki: Kawa no Soku-Heki (river side-wall) and *Kawa no Zoko* (river bottom)

The river's sides and bottom, referred to in the Japanese lexicon respectively as *kawa no soku-heki* and *kawa no zoko*, are the structures/concepts from the river metaphor that stand for the client's environment. These are perhaps the most important determinants of a person's life flow in a collectivist social context because of the primacy afforded to the environmental context in determining the experiences of self and subsequent meanings of personal action. In the Kawa model, the river walls and sides represent the subject's social and physical contexts. The social context comprises mainly those who share a direct relationship with the subject. Depending upon which social frame is perceived as being most important in a given instance and place, the riversides and bottom can represent family members, pets (dearly loved and appreciated companions with whom people develop profoundly meaningful relationships), workmates, friends in a recreational club, classmates, etc. Deceased family members or friends whose memory exerts an influence on meanings in a person's or group's daily life, can and should be included here.

Conversing with deceased loved ones might qualify a person for a psychiatric consult in a certain cultural interpretation of normal, but in the framework of the Kawa model, this can represent a legitimate human occupation. In certain non-Western societies, like those of Japan, social relationships are regarded to be the central[5] determinant, of individual and collective life flow.

Aspects of the surrounding social frame on the subject can affect the overall flow (volume and rate) of the *kawa*. Harmonious relationships can enable and complement life flow. Increased flow can have an agent effect upon difficult circumstances and problems as the force of water displaces rocks in the channel and even create new courses through which to flow. Conversely, a decrease in flow volume can exert a compounding, negative effect on the other elements that take up space in the channel (Figure 7.4). If there are obstructions (rocks and driftwood) in the watercourse when river walls and bottom are thickened and constricting, the flow of the river is especially compromised. As we will see, the rocks in this river can directly butt up against the river walls and bottom, compounding and creating larger impediments to the river's usual flow. When applying the Kawa model in collectivist-oriented populations, these components and the perceptions of their importance are paramount.

Like all other elements of the river, these concepts are always interpreted in relation to the whole, taking into consideration all other elements of the subject's context and their interrelations/interdependencies. Occupational

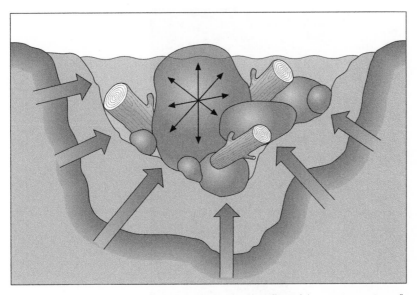

Figure 7.4 Cross-section view of a client's Kawa showing the effect of river components on flow.

therapists have traditionally been concerned with a 'holistic' view of the client. Most therapists would be concerned if his or her role was limited in practice scope to assessing and treating pathology. Occupational therapists have long appreciated and concerned themselves with the social consequences affecting the client's ability to engage in functional and meaningful daily activities resulting from a particular pathology.

Iwa (rocks)

Iwa (Japanese for large rocks or crags) represent discrete circumstances that are considered to be impediments to one's *life flow*. They are life circumstances perceived by the client to be problematic and difficult to remove. Most rivers, like people's lives, have such rocks or impediments, of varying size, shape and number. Large rocks, by themselves or in combination with other rocks, jammed directly or indirectly against the river walls and sides (environment) can profoundly impede and obstruct flow. The client's rocks may have been there since the beginning, such as with congenital conditions. They may appear instantaneously, as in sudden illness or injury, and even be transient. If you reflect on your own life as a river, you may see a variety of rocks (of different sizes and shapes) in your river. Some of these rocks remain unremarkable until they butt up against certain aspects of the social and physical environment.

The impeding effect of rocks can compound when situated against the river's sides and walls (environment). A person's bodily impairment becomes disabling when interfaced with the environment. For example, the functional difficulties associated with a neurological condition can change according to the environmental context. A (physically) barrier-free environment can decrease one's disability, as can social and/or political/organisational environments that are accepting and accommodating of people with disabling conditions.

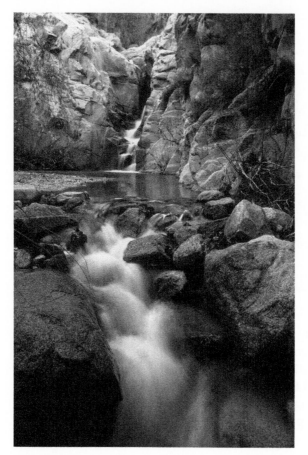

Figure 7.5 Rocks (Iwa)

Auditory hallucinations become even more problematic in a congested social environment; sexual orientation can become more of a discouraging issue for a person in the context of a hostile and intolerant social context; being unable to walk becomes a problem when the laws do not require workplaces to be accessible by wheelchair; sexual impotence may be less of a problem until it involves a sexual partner (social environment).

Once the client's perceived rocks are known (including their relative size and situation), the therapist can help to identify potential areas of intervention and strategies to enable better life flow. The broader contextual definition of disabling circumstances necessarily brings into play the client's surrounding environment. Occupational therapy intervention can therefore include treatment strategies that expand beyond the traditional medical patient, to his or her social network and even to policies and social structures that ultimately play a part in setting the disabling context.

How are the problems, in your current practice, to which you are mandated to address as an occupational therapist defined? What are the cultural boundaries that inform your current scope of practice and is this satisfactory to you? Occupational therapy has always been, in its contemporary practice, about meeting the client's needs in the context of their daily living. The Kawa model may assist the therapist in visioning the relationship between the client(s) and their context and help to clarify the targets of a more holistic occupational therapy practice.

The subject, be it an individual or a collective, ideally determines the specific rocks, their number, magnitude, form and situation in the river. As with all other elements of the model, if the client is unable to express their own river, family members or a community of people connected with the issue at hand may lend assistance. Often, it is the probing questions that follow that provide better and specific insights into the quality of the water flow around certain *iwa*. Upon viewing one of the client's rocks sitting against a thickened wall of the river, the therapist may ask the client: 'What is this rock and what kinds of problems is it creating in your social life or environment?'

Ryuboku (Driftwood)

Ryuboku is Japanese for 'driftwood', and represents the subject's personal attributes and resources, such as values (i.e. honesty, thrift), character (i.e. optimism, stubbornness), personality (i.e. reserved, outgoing), special skill (i.e. carpentry, public speaking), immaterial (i.e. friends, siblings) and material (i.e. wealth, special equipment) assets and living situation (rural and urban, shared accommodations, etc) that can positively or negatively affect the subject's circumstance and life flow.

Like driftwood they are transient in nature and carry a certain quality of fate or serendipity. They can appear to be inconsequential in some instances and significantly obstructive in others – particularly when they settle in among

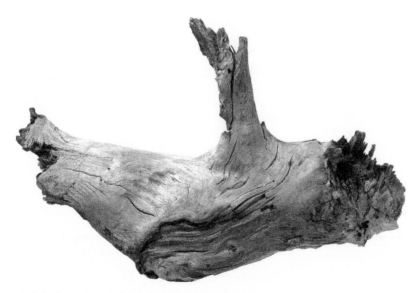

Figure 7.6 Driftwood (Ryuboku)

rocks and the river sides and walls. On the other hand, they can collide with the same structures to nudge obstructions out of the way. A client's religious faith and sense of determination can be positive factors in persevering to erode or move rocks out of the way. Receiving a grant to acquire specialised assistive equipment can turn out to be the piece of driftwood that collides against existing flow impediments and opens a greater channel for one's life to flow more strongly. Traditionally, many of these matters were treated from an individual perspective and in genres of research, such as psychology, these were treated more as individual embodiments rather than being located both inside the human being as well as in the environmental realm. Once again, the attitude demonstrated in this rendition of the Kawa model here is that human phenomena and the ascription of meaning occur both inside and outside of the human body, in a broader, integrated frame. In the Japanese occupational therapy experience the practice norm has been to reflect the occurrence of driftwood in the Kawa model drawings to the client and allow them to speak to the driftwood's location and function from their perspective.

Table 7.1 gives some examples of what *ryuboku* might look like and their consequent effects on a client's life flow at a particular place in time.

Driftwood is a part of everyone's river and is often those intangible components possessed by each unique client of occupational therapy. Effective therapists pay particular attention to these components of a client's or community's assets and circumstances, and consider their real or potential effect on the client's situation. Should a particular client issue be depicted by an *iwa*, *torimaki*, or *ryuboku*? It is important for the client to place their issues in a particular category. Regardless of which category an issue is placed in, its relation to other structures/factors/issues and the dynamics that accompany

TABLE 7.1 SUMMARY OF DRIFTWOOD EFFECT EXAMPLES		
Ryuboku / driftwood	**Positive effect (+)**	**Negative effect (−)**
Future expectations	Goals, something to look forward to	A source of frustration, stress, worry
Parent's financial status	Help with equipment, home renovations	Increased dependency, lack of skill development
Stubbornness	Determination to succeed	Source of frustration
Substance abuse (alcoholism)	Social network at the pub	Decreased motivation, initiative
Bipolar mood swings	Sense of well-being and confidence	Sense of despair and decreased energy
Moving to city	Convenience and access to special programmes, anonymity	Lack of support, new stresses

An Overview of the Kawa Model

its placement are the most important considerations. In some situations, depending on social cultural norms, as we will see in the next chapter, the occupational therapist may be the one to draw the river. The therapist in these cases will attempt to interpret the client(s)' narratives and derive a river diagram to use as a common metaphor for dialogue. The aim is to arrive at a mutual understanding of the client's experience of well-being and disablement and the rich surrounding context that gives these issues their quality and meaning. In other situations, it will be the client or community that will configure their river. Ideally the identification, quality and placement of the river components will be determined through a dialogue between all parties involved. The most accurate depiction of the client's context, as the client sees things, will lead to the most meaningful and effective interventions.

Expertise becomes apparent in the therapist's decisions regarding when to enhance or de-emphasise the effect of particular driftwood.

Sukima (Space between Obstructions) Where Life Energy Still Flows: The Promise of Occupational Therapy

Now that the purpose of the metaphor of a river to depict a person's life flow and situation is clearer, attention can be focused on the *sukima* (spaces between the rocks, driftwood, and river walls and bottom). These spaces are as important to comprehend in the client as are the other elements of the river when determining how to apply and direct occupational therapy. In the Kawa model, spaces are the points through which the client's life energy (water) evidently flows. In an extreme sense, these are those factors that sustain the client's hope of seeing a new day. For example, a space between a functional impairment such as arthritis (an *iwa*/rock) and a social group or person (in the river sides and walls) may represent a certain social role, such as parent, company worker, friend, etc.

The spaces through which life flows, is representative of 'occupation', from an Eastern perspective.

Water naturally coursing through these spaces can work to erode the rocks and river walls and bottom and over time transform them into larger conduits for life flow (Figure 7.8). This effect reflects the latent healing potential that each subject naturally holds within themselves and in the inseparable context. Thus, occupational therapy in this perspective retains its hallmark of working with the client's abilities and assets. It also directs occupational therapy intervention towards all elements (in this case a medically defined problem, various aspects and levels of environment) in the context.

Spaces, then, represent important foci for occupational therapy. They occur throughout the context of the self and environs; between the rocks, walls and

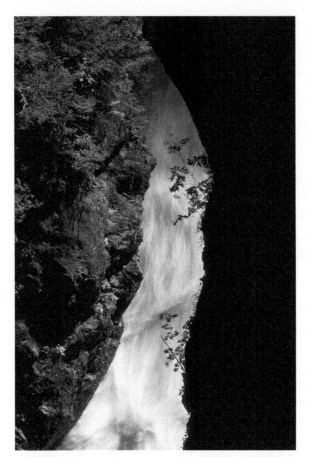

Figure 7.7 Spaces (Sukima)

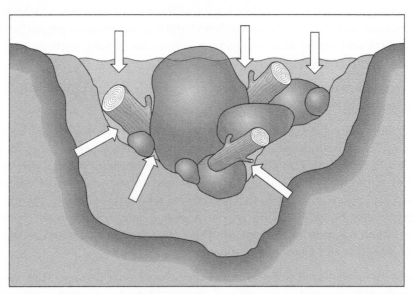

Figure 7.8 Cross-sectional view of several gaps in the client's Kawa pointing to potential targets for occupational therapy interventions.

bottom, and driftwood. Spaces subsume the environment as part of the greater context of the problem and expand the scope of intervention to integrate naturally what, in the Western sense, would have been treated separately through the dualism of internal (pertaining to *self* and personal attributes) and external (environment constructed as separate and outside of the self). *Spaces* are potential channels for the client's flow, allowing client and therapist to determine multiple points and levels of intervention (Figure 7.9). In this way, each problem or enabling opportunity is bounded by and appreciated in a broader context.

The concepts and the contextual application of the Kawa model are by natural design, flexible and adaptable. Each client's unique river takes its important concepts and configuration from the situation of the subject, in a given time and place. The definition of problems and circumstances are broad – as broad and diverse as our clients' worlds of meanings. In turn, this particular conceptualisation of people and their circumstances foreshadows the broad outlook and scope of occupational therapy interventions, when set in particular cultural contexts.

Rather than attempting to reduce a person's problems (i.e. focusing only on rocks) to discrete issues, isolated out of their particular contexts, similar to the rational processes in which client problems are identified and discretely named/diagnosed in conventional Western health practice, the Kawa model framework compels the occupational therapist to view and treat issues within a holistic framework, seeking to appreciate the clients' identified issues within their integrated, inseparable contexts. Occupation is therefore regarded in wholes, to include the meaning of the activity to self and community to

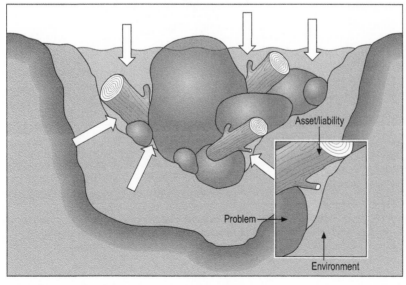

Figure 7.9 Cross-sectional view of a gap in the client's Kawa pointing to the importance of understanding the client's context to set priorities for occupational therapy.

which the individual inseparably belongs, and not just in terms of biomechanical components, or individually embodied and defined pathology and function.

Phenomena and life circumstances rarely occur in isolation. By changing one aspect of the client's world, all other aspects of his or her river change. The river's spaces represent opportunities to problem solve and focus therapy on positive opportunities, which may have little direct relation to the person's medically defined condition.

By using this model, occupational therapists, in partnership with their clients, are directed to stem further obstruction of life energy/flow and look for every opportunity in the broader context, to enhance it (Figure 7.10). Occupational therapy is reconceptualised to mean enabling life energy or life flow. Life is like a river. The volume, rate and quality of its flow determine, and are determined by, the constellation of factors that comprise the inseparable person–environment relationship. The quality of flow is disrupted, altered, and even catastrophically slowed, as normal occurrences in life.

'What is occupation, and what do occupational therapists do?' In some cultures, clients may understand: 'Occupation is life flow and occupational therapists are enablers of people's life flow', better than the standard textbook definitions that we all learned as students.

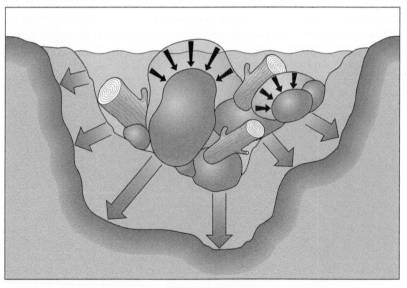

Figure 7.10 Cross-sectional view of a client's Kawa. Occupational therapists, in partnership with their clients, are directed to stem further obstruction of life energy/flow and look for every opportunity, in the broader context, to enhance and maximise the client's life flow.

REFERENCES

[1] Okuda M, Kataoka N, Takahashi H, et al. The Kawa (River) Model: Reflections on Our Culture. Singapore: 3rd Asia Pacific Occupational Therapy Congress; 2003

[2] Lakoff G, Johnson M. Metaphors We Live By. Chicago: University of Chicago Press; 1980

[3] Lebra TS. Japanese Patterns of Behavior. Honolulu: University of Hawaii Press; 1976

[4] Doi T. The Anatomy of Dependence. Tokyo: Kodansha International; 1973

[5] Nakane C. Tate shakai no ningen kankei [Human Relations in a Vertical Society]. Tokyo: Kodansha; 1970

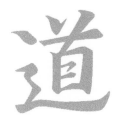

CHAPTER 8

Applying the Kawa Model

Comprehending Occupation in Context

道

How do you presently apply occupational therapy theory to practice? Do you follow a particular protocol, like a recipe, assuming that the model, its concepts and principles adequately reflect and represent the client's view of reality and shared meanings of occupations in daily life? Some occupational therapists have abandoned conceptual models and theory altogether, thinking they are too abstract and lacking in relevance to what actually happens in that interface between therapist and client. Perhaps therapists' resistance to using theory has something to do with learning difficult concepts, as if learning a new model carries the challenge of learning a new language without any guarantees that the language and the ideas it translates can be understood by clients (and occupational therapists). Or perhaps there is a growing sense of frustration that even if the theoretical material is relevant to the client, the institutional conditions and policies of the facilities and contexts in which occupational therapists practise ultimately determine how much of a particular theory can be utilised. For these and many other reasons, a certain dissonance for theory seems to have formed, resulting in its dismissal – as something to be studied and left in the halls of occupational therapy professional entry programmes.

One of the possible reasons for theory's demise as described may be found in the genesis and dynamics of theory development prevalent in the fields of applied health professions. Theory has traditionally been a 'top-down' approach in which one or several theorists think about a better way to describe what they believe they see, and postulate or hypothesise an explanation. This *cultural* tradition is the one that has been handed down through the scientific method and carries certain tacit assumptions. One such assumption is that the explanation of a given phenomenon that theory yields is universal. Good or valid theory in this regard is meant to stand the rigour of systematic testing, and graduate from merely a set of (someone's) ideas (or postulates), to a more credible, believable set of principles – or laws. Unfortunately, one cannot always transfer these procedures that have served science well for describing and explaining physical objects and phenomena to matters of social phenomena and culture. We have come to the thinking that our social behaviour patterns, including occupation (whatever it may mean) and the meanings ascribed to agency are not universally wired into our DNA. Explanations for why people do what they do and the meanings that are ascribed to them are still being discoursed in the social sciences. However, the leanings of the thesis presented in this book are towards the understanding that the meanings of people's actions vary according to *culture*. That is, according to shared spheres of common experience, situated in a particular place and time.

Conventional models carry through their top-down structure of genesis into their applications with clients in occupational therapy. We may claim to be enacting client-centred practice, yet the clients' narratives are ultimately reduced, organised and made sense of through the structure, language and explanatory principles of our professional models and theory. This is even more so the case when proprietary measurement instruments that are tied to a particular model are being implemented with strict dedication to following protocol under the pretence of scientific rigour.

The genesis and development of the Kawa model followed the antithesis to the top-down dynamic, in beginning with no universal assumptions about what occupational therapy was or what it meant to its clientele. There was a founding belief that the meaning and mysteries around these and other meanings of occupational therapy were embedded in the social contexts of occupational therapists and their clients, waiting to be uncovered, brought into view and appreciated. The structure, concepts and principles of this new conceptual model would emerge out of the real day-to-day experiences and explanations of real people. And herein lies the essence of the Kawa model's application. In a similar way in which the Kawa model was raised from the bottom up, the client's narrative is illuminated and made central. The client will actually name his or her own concepts and explain the principles that tie these concepts together in the rigour of his or her own cultural lens.

Principles of Use

As we proceed to think about applying the Kawa model in our own practices, there are several points to consider. Throughout this work, culture has been defined in a broader sense, simply as 'shared spheres of meanings', from a cultural relativist or social constructionist perspective, and this holds fundamental sway in how the model is intended to be interpreted and applied.

Universalistic and Particularistic Views of Reality: Honouring the Client and Trusting Emergence

The first point to consider is that all universalistic assumptions regarding the relevance and explanatory power of this model are to be discarded. This may be difficult to do, as many of us may have become used to projecting our own views of reality and proper ways of acting onto others – even onto people who have grown through other, different spheres of experience than our own. If the model and the metaphor on which it is based fail to resonate or hold appropriate meaning to either the client or occupational therapist, it should be modified or placed aside in exchange for a more relevant and appropriate model. The client's narrative becomes *the model* on which the promise of occupational therapy as an enabling force is reconciled. Bernard Glaser[1], one of the founders of grounded theory methodology in the qualitative research genre stated the phrase: 'trust emergence'. In applying the Kawa model, the occupational therapist has to become used to trusting that the client's narrative will emerge through a process of enabling him or her to do so.

Another point then to keep in mind, is to be aware of your own 'cultural lens'. The occupational therapist should realise that his or her own interpretations of reality, including making sense of and appreciating the client, occur through a kind of filter that is informed by one's own spheres of shared experiences. Not only does cultural situation concern the meanings of objects and phenomena, but also the structure of social norms that govern, shape and reflect meaning in the structure and content of human interactions. The competent therapist will not only appreciate the culture embodied in the client, but also the cultures at play within one's self, within the occupational therapy as you have learned and experienced it, and the institutional conditions that set the structure and mandate for the therapeutic process. This is not a simple undertaking, by any means, but a good place to start is simply being aware of the existence of such contexts and being vigilant about the influences and potential effects of these respective cultural contexts.

Centralised and Decentralised Self: Balance, Control and Harmony

How one constructs the world and situates one's 'self' in relation has had fundamental bearing on the conceptualisations and meanings of occupation. The interpretations and meanings of what people do in the world may vary according to whether the *self* is believed to be situated in a central privileged position vis-à-vis a discrete, separate environment[2,3], or is believed to be merely one integrated part of a greater universe (*no less than the trees and the stars*[4]). Alternate, competing world views and *self* construal, which surely exists among a diverse occupational therapy clientele, challenges the universal premise of conventional occupational therapy models. These models assume a centrally situated *self*, separated[5,2] from a surrounding, discrete environment that one 'occupies' through rational, purposeful, action or 'doing'. Well-being coincides with balance between *self* and one's environs. Balance in this sense is not necessarily the kind of equilibrium indicated by 'zero' on a weigh scale but rather a state in which a privileged *self* is able to exploit the environment and exercise control over his or her perceived circumstances. With this particular *self*-agency comes a sense of entitlement to doing in the present that extends temporally into the future. We not only expect to control our immediate circumstances, but also set future objectives in an attempt to control our own destinies. It should come as little surprise, then, to see that independence, autonomy, egalitarianism, and self-determinism, are celebrated ideals that point to a common world view and value pattern shared between mainstream occupational therapy ideology and the wider Western social context that raised it [2]. The Kawa model departs from this construal of a centrally situated and agent self. Applied to client contexts in its original form, the lines between self and environment and context are blurred. They are all treated as integrated parts of a whole frame. Thus, the entire diagram of the river illustrates the self embedded in the environment and circumstance. And occupation is comprehended in this context.

Another point to keep in mind is the treatment of time or temporal orientation. In a holistic regard for the world and self, as illustrated in the East Asian variation of the cosmological myth, temporal orientation tends to be sensed in the here-and-now as neither the past nor the future are considered products. A state of wellness coincides when all elements in a frame, including the self, coexist in harmony. This harmony is the sought-after *balance* in the river-life metaphor, and disruption of this harmony hampers the collective synergy or life flow/energy (Figure 8.1). The thought of 'enhancing or restoring harmony' supplanting 'enabling unilateral control' as a primary purpose for occupational therapy may represent a restoration of familiar views of health in many non-Western contexts. In mainstream Western contexts, such harmony may represent a new way to think about client issues of balance and control. In light of these varied interpretations of occupation and well-being matters of occupational balance ought to re-examined from a broader cultural perspective.

This construction of *harmony* – a state of individual or collective being in which the subject, be it self or community, is in *balance* with the context that it is a part of forms the underlying ontology of the Kawa/river framework. The essence of this harmony is conceptualised as 'life-energy' or 'life flow'. Occupational therapy's purpose is to help the subject enhance and balance this flow. In this balance, there is coexistence – a synergy between all elements of the river. The symbolic meanings of rocks, river walls and sides, driftwood and water, combine to form the profound context that affects flow. While the occupational therapist is working out the shape, content and configuration of the river metaphor with the client(s), he or she will be aware of the following issues represented by these questions: 'How can one come to terms with one's circumstances? How can harmony between the elements, of which *one* is merely one part, be realised? How and in what way can occupational therapy assist the processes and enable greater flow?'

Occupational therapy issues, from this holistic regard, are represented by a complex interplay of self and context. Occupational therapy solutions through the Kawa metaphor, likewise, involve all of these elements in the frame.

Application

What do all of the previous stated principles suggest about how the model should be used and applied in occupational therapy processes? All of these points underscore the premise that there is not one 'right' way to use and apply the Kawa model. The Kawa is a metaphor for life. The *right* way is realised when the model is adapted and used as a vehicle to illuminate the client's narrative for his or her life at a certain place and point in time. The Kawa model's ultimate form will be determined by the unique qualities of

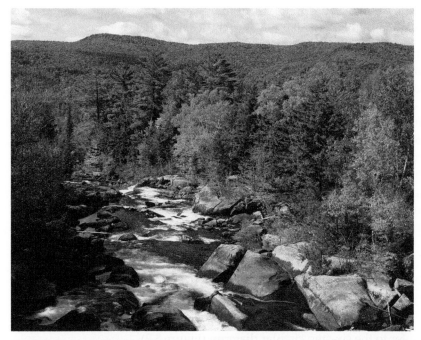

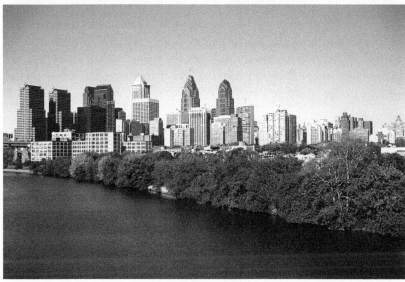

Figure 8.1 What constitutes a state of balance and harmony in a person's life is personally and culturally specific. Each of these rivers or life flows can represent the ideal or optimal regard for daily life.

the client and the occupational therapy frame. In this following section, a generic protocol is offered, with the premise that the Kawa model is not a universally applicable framework. The model was originally developed in Japanese contexts and has its own particular application protocols in Japanese contexts. However, occupational therapists around the world have tested the model in a variety of cultural and social contexts and have experienced

163

favourable results concerning its utility – especially when adapted and changed to meet the particular needs of the local culture.

In each varying setting, the model and metaphor have been modified and interpreted in varying ways. Unlike conventional theory application, occupational therapists are encouraged to evaluate critically the effectiveness of the Kawa model and alter it to suit the therapeutic frame. The bottom line for evaluating whether the model is useful or not will be the degree to which the client agrees on the model's ability to represent his or her narrative of well-being and day-to-day experience of life. If the model falls short of this criterion, the therapist should seriously consider discarding the model or altering the model to make it suitable and culturally safe. The Kawa model is not a universal conceptual model and therefore can be altered suitably to meet the needs of the client and occupational therapist.

Suggested Steps towards Using the Model in Clinical Practice Situations

Please refer to the six-step circular diagram (Figure 8.2).

These are merely suggested steps. In keeping with the relational qualities and the philosophical bases for the Kawa model, occupational therapists should explore various and creative ways for utilising the Kawa model. Therapists are then encouraged to share their experiences and insights on the Kawa model forum (website under construction).

Step One: Who Is the Client?

The first step involves determining whether the Kawa (river) metaphor resonates in meaning with the client (and the occupational therapist, of course) and therefore whether the Kawa model is appropriate to use in this situation. Additional comments and discussion of who (a person or collective) or what (organisations, communities, processes such as rehabilitation team mandates, etc.) the client is and who actually draws the river diagram are commented on in the section immediately following.

If the client is an individual and has the capability to reveal aspects of his or her daily life experience and circumstance, invite him or her to draw a picture or diagram of a river to depict his current state of being or circumstance. This may start off with a simple explanation like: 'Would you mind drawing a picture of a river?' This can then be followed by: 'Suppose this river is your life at this point in time, can you continue your drawing to make it represent your present situation?' The opportunity exists to use this process to develop a dialogue between client and occupational therapist that allows the therapist a

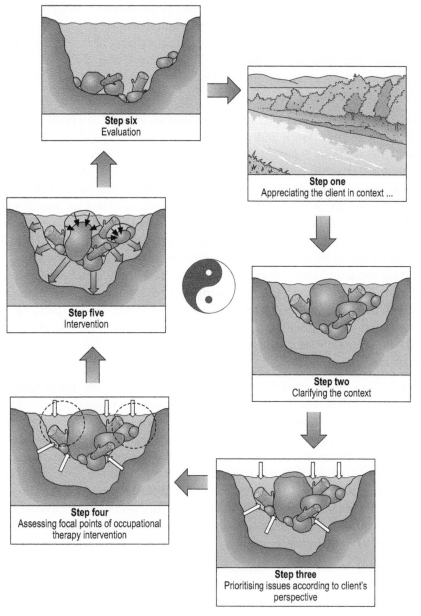

Figure 8.2 A suggested six-step approach in employing the Kawa model in occupational therapy practice contexts.

more profound view and appreciation for the client's life circumstance and context, in the client's own words and descriptions of the circumstances. Mental health workers have commented that the river model exercise has afforded them a more comprehensive view into the delusional qualities of the client with schizophrenia. The delusions may be dismissed by the professional as non-real, but they constitute major factors that are *real* and problematic to the client. Remember, the Kawa is a metaphor of the client's view of reality and circumstance, and for this reason, it is important to trust emergence[1] and seize the opportunity to see the issues as accurately as possible from the client's viewpoint and contexts of meaning. The occupational therapist will be afforded the privilege to comprehend what *occupation* might really look like and mean to the client.

Through a process of dialogue, structures that are present can be discussed in terms of their importance and relevance to the client. The client can also be asked whether there is anything missing in the river diagram. It is up to the occupational therapist then to talk about the component of the formal model, such as the rocks, river side walls, driftwood and water courses. You may choose to say, for example: 'If rocks of various sizes stand for problems or challenges that sit in your river and block or slow down the water flowing, what would they be … can you draw them into your river?' This particular discussion might be followed by a suggestion that the river walls and floor stand for social and physical environment, such as family members and living situation. This discussion might be furthered by a frank discussion about if and how the problems are intertwined and how these problems (pain, limited motor function, cognitive deficits, etc.) or challenges interface and impact the social environment (family members) or physical environment (apartment or workplace).

Though the original model conceptualised 'driftwood', the client may use other forms of debris or 'pollution' to name transient, yet significant, modifiers of water flow. Instead of driftwood, the object may be 'an old tyre' or 'a bicycle lying twisted and jammed against the rocks'. The client might subsequently explain that: 'Since my relapse, I cannot drive anymore'; or 'My hopes of making the Olympic trials were erased when that car hit me'. One of the keys through this whole process is to enable the client to express their situation freely and to use the opportunity to verify, affirm, probe deeper and explore the interrelations of the constellation of factors that make up the client's experience of daily living.

This exercise is not about accuracy or aesthetics, though the exercise can serve other alternate functional performance assessment. Dexterity, neuro-psychological performance, visual spatial and other cognitive performance function, sitting tolerance, etc., are some examples of alternate evaluation of client performance that have been anecdotally reported to the author by occupational therapists trialling this model in diverse practice settings.

The level of insight that the client has into their situation may be an especial factor during this beginning phase. In Asian cultural settings, for example, the rational and individual-centric exercise of reflection and self-insight may be challenging. With the primary aim being to derive as best a 'picture' of the client's narrative, the therapist can decide to include other members of the client's social network. Japanese therapists, for example, have commented on how useful the Kawa model is in enabling a discussion of concern for the client's situation. A conference attended by supportive, loving family members that focuses on making sure that the client's context of experiences around a disabling issue is comprehensively understood, are the seeds to a preferred outcome. The end result of such a process can be a more effective occupational therapy with accurate and meaningful targets for occupational and health team intervention. A rich and comprehensive appreciation of the client in the context of day-to-day experiences and meanings, derived in a relatively short time, is possible through the Kawa model. In individual application situations, if the level of insight possible is less than useful, the therapist should continue with the model's application. Over time, occupational therapists using the Kawa model report that the Kawa becomes more familiar and less threatening, to yield diagrams demonstrating greater, more comprehensive insights into a client's situation.

Because the Kawa metaphor is easy to comprehend and familiarity with its use by both therapist and client develops with frequency, occupational therapists will discover their own ways to use it. Whether the structure, concepts and inner dynamics are interpreted differently and subsequently altered or the frequency of use changes, the model *should* be altered to make it relevant to your practice context. Western occupational therapists, oriented more rationally, may prefer to implement the model at least three times in a particular client's case. Using one Kawa diagram and discussion around the client's current situation, one Kawa diagram and discussion around the client's situation in the past (before the current circumstances transpired), and one Kawa diagram set in the client's future to speculate where and what kind of state he or she envisions, appears to be a use pattern that is emerging. Unlike other contemporary conceptual models, the Kawa model appears to be unique in this longitudinal application.

The Kawa drawings should not be discarded, as the issues and points for occupational therapy intervention identified through each rendition of the drawings will serve as a record of progress over time.

Creative additions to the Kawa model and its evolution as a useful tool internationally and inter-culturally are welcomed and encouraged.

Step Two: Clarify the Context

Clarifying, and comprehensively understanding, the client's metaphorical representations, of his or her *occupational* circumstances, represents the second step. Like an artist coming back to an original painting and applying the final brush-strokes to achieve a satisfactory representation of an internally held image, this is the stage at which the dialogue in the therapeutic relationship is focused on the quality of the symbolic representations of the client's world of meanings. This entails questions and queries to affirm the meaning of the magnitudes, relative locations and relationships between the objects that make up the client's river. 'What is this rock here, and why is this one so big?' 'This rock is wedged between these other two large rocks and all three are resting against this part of the river wall … why?' The client may decide to change the drawing by altering the number, shape, texture and placement of the various parts of the river.

Although the emphasis so far has been on assessment, this dialogue of affirming and clarifying can be a therapeutic activity in itself. New insights are uncovered and a dialogue about possible solutions is enabled. The interrelatedness of all objects and phenomena in a particular frame is made explicit, and the complexities of the context around the client's occupational issues are raised into view. The therapeutic relationship is strengthened here as the depth of the occupational therapist's interest in the client's circumstances is progressed. This is the beginning of the enabling process, and the quality of trust and cooperation established between the therapist and client sets the stage for the processes that follow.

Step Three: Prioritising Issues According to the Client's Perspective

This is a continuation of the previous stage with a new dimension coming into view – occupational therapy. Between the rocks, river sides and walls and driftwood/debris, where the water continues to flow, there lies potential for positive development and change. Put in a different way, between the client's identified problems and challenges, personal assets and liabilities, transient factors, and environmental factors (social, including political and institutional, and physical), lie potential courses and channels through which a person's life continues to flow. These spaces and channels symbolise the potential applications and the enabling power of occupational therapy. At this step, those potential spaces are located and identified. The boundaries of the spaces – their size and shape – are ascertained through the ongoing reflective dialogue between client and therapist. The structures that bound the spaces and weak spots are explored further with the client, giving greater and more profound insights into the complexities and context surrounding these points. 'Decreasing pain', or 'increasing range of motion', for example, which are typical medical and biomechanically oriented points of interest, appear overly simple and almost never emerge in such a unidimensional form in a Kawa analysis. Rather, such simplistic points are replaced by more complex, multidimensional descriptions of a client's *occupational* circumstance, which almost always entail an environmental and a client-embodied facet.

Whenever a medically defined problem is expressed (usually by a 'rock'), it is usually expressed in concert with the social consequences that interface with it (river side or bottom). Hence, the occupational therapist should probe these relationships further to gain a more comprehensive understanding of the quality of an identified occupational issue. As in other functional assessment phases, the thoroughness of the inquiry leading to a more accurate description of the problem(s) will have a profound effect upon the effectiveness of the occupational therapy process that follows.

The occupational therapist should not limit his or her search for potential occupational therapy intervention points to spaces and gaps that appear between rocks, driftwood and the river walls and floor. The process of identifying potential points in a dialogue with the client should also include weaknesses where gaps might be created. For example, a completely closed seam (dependency) between a rock, like a person's congenital disability and the river bottom – his parent's unwillingness for him to move out of the family home – could easily be looked over during a therapist's search for potential intervention sites. This closed seam might be opened to allow some life to flow through by eroding the rock (perhaps by enabling the client to acquire independent living skills) and eroding the river bottom (by conferring with the parents to advocate for their son's quest to leave home). It is important that the client partners with the occupational therapist in determining the location, methods and timing and planning of the mutually derived interventions. The therapist must exercise superior imagination, creativity, a positive regard for the client's potential, and the specialised knowledge set acquired in professional training to practise occupational therapy in the framework of the Kawa model.

Eventually, these spaces or potential points for occupational therapy intervention will be further assessed and prioritised. Once again, this will be a process that will ideally involve both client and therapist.

Step Four: Assessing Focal Points of Occupational Therapy Intervention

Once the potential targets for occupational therapy intervention are identified in the client's river, the occupational therapist and client engage in a process of quantifying the magnitude, and ascertaining the quality of the various structures involved. The therapist may choose to use a selection of established instruments in concert with qualitative methods to acquire a more objective sense of the nature and magnitude of the points of occupational therapy intervention. If the process has progressed well, the client will continue to hold a primary role in his or her treatment. The Kawa model provides an organising framework and situates the identified problems in a metaphor that is easy to visualise and reconcile to the client's sphere of meanings. The intervention points are real, named in the client's lexicon, fundamentally meaningful and directly involve the client's active participation.

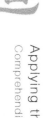

Step Five: Intervention

Now that the channels through which the client's life energy flow are identified, including the contextual factors that shape and border them, and prioritised with the client, the intervention can be planned and implemented. Occupational therapists will have noticed by this stage of the model's use that many of the occupational issues identified are not part of the usual occupational therapy mandate set by institutions and traditional rehabilitation treatment protocols. For one thing, the identified challenges and issues are specific and uniquely configured to individual context and the client's meanings ascribed to them. It may be frustrating to the therapist (and client groups) to come to the realisation that institutional mandates are usually drawn, despite the best intentions, through a medical cultural lens and thus accountable to outcome measures and factors that appeal to medical, economical and political oriented interests and not necessarily to mandates and outcomes that are most meaningful to the client. The Kawa model may help the occupational therapist see, appreciate and illuminate the occupational issues and occupational consequences of the client's medically defined problems. In a middle Western context, conceptual models like the Canadian Model of Occupational Performance (CMOP)[6] and the Model of Human Occupation (MOHO)[7] perform this function admirably. Culturally relevant occupational therapy models can inform and equip the therapist with useful frameworks to make sense of the client's occupational issues in the face of biomedicine's awesome explanatory power.

Intervention approaches are as complex, effective, unique and meaningful as the original framing of the client's issues in context. In using the Kawa model, a multi-faceted approach is taken, as all of the factors that bind and give shape to a particular water channel are fair game when selecting the target points and methods for intervention. The basic premise of intervention, conveyed through the river metaphor, is the channelling and focusing of water pressure (the client's residual abilities and skills) on the target points of intervention. The action may be to erode the surface of a rock or river wall, push rocks out of the way, breaking rocks and other structures through water force (life force and determination), push driftwood away or against another problematic structure to smash the impediment or move it out of the way.

A client's decreased participation in community life of watching the game on the television at the local public house while lifting a pint with his pals, may be bound by his decreased standing tolerance (rock), decreased confidence and self-image (driftwood), inaccessible facilities (river wall) and a concerned and over-protective spouse (river bottom). In this example, the occupational therapist might consider: activities that simulate and enhance standing tolerance during occupational therapy; grade occupational therapy activities with aim to support client's sense of ability and achievement; advocate to the proprietor of the public house regarding the client's wish to access; and arrange a conference with the family to discuss support and enablement of the client to engage in this important activity.

Depending on priority of intervention, the client and therapist may work on activities that address several identified problems referring to different frames/water channels, simultaneously. In concert with the natural river metaphor, which mirrors the East Asian cosmological myth, the therapist should keep in mind that change in the broader context is never isolated. Everything is interconnected and integrated. When change is introduced in any point in the context, all other parts of the whole are affected and also subject to change. This is the synergy of the integrated, inseparable whole. Like a river that changes as a result of a rock falling into it, even though imperceptive when viewed from the surface, the inner shape, configuration and hydrodynamics are significantly altered. A person's restored ability to toilet independently, in a particular context, may boost his confidence and sense of well-being, indirectly increasing his abilities in other performance areas and in his disposition and social interactions. Rehabilitation professionals working in health facilities have experienced this integrative synergy in their practices, despite the conventional rational medical approaches that tend to reduce the complexities and integrative nature of human well-being.

The power of occupational therapy lies in the relevance of its ideas and practices to the complex, dynamic, real, day-to-day experiences of ordinary people ... like a river.

Step Six: Evaluation

Acknowledgement of the uniqueness and the particular nature of the client's patterns, forms, meanings and experiences, etc. of occupation tightly integrated in a particular context, holds significant implications for evaluating client progress and outcomes. For this Kawa client-centred view entails a client-centred measurement criterion. This is a departure somewhat from the conventional view of the client being evaluated against some externally located standard or narrative that often accompanies a universal representation of 'normal'. One can gather by now that a constructionist view of human agency questions just what *normal* means – the grand goal of independence in self-care and activities of daily living, supported by values that espouse autonomy, self-efficacy and individual determinism, etc. These Western-centric norms are lost on people who have been raised in collectivist cultures where the norm is closer to ideals on interdependence and harmony with nature and circumstance.

The Kawa model starts with the client's introspective view of his or her own occupational situation and ends with the same. (The client, of course, is not limited to an individual but can relate to a collective.) The usual practice of measuring a person's performance against some external criterion is replaced by the practice of measuring or evaluating the client's performance against his or her own criteria. This can be accomplished by simply comparing drawings and explanations of one's river chronologically. 'When we first started off, your river was looking quite "busy" and the water flow was blocked up heavily in a number of places. What is different in this newest drawing of your river?' An important dialogue can be enabled in which the various targets of intervention, spanning the client and his or her surrounding context, are brought into view and analysed by both client and therapist. Of course, client and therapist are never bound to the Kawa metaphor. One might begin with the Kawa metaphor and use it only as a framework to organise the dialogue and occupational therapy process, then move to a specific issue or problem identified and take it from there. Ultimately, the client's narrative of his or her account of occupational being is important to comprehend, being the basis from which the entire occupational therapy process is configured.

Once again, what might be construed as a process of assessment, can also function as intervention. The discussion can broach the topic of what went better, what did not change and what aspects of the client's flow worsened. There is an opportunity to explore mutually the reasons for progress or regression, and what may have transpired over the brief time since the last drawing of the river. Westerners applying the model may emphasise the rational perspective in taking control of one's river and may choose to identify factors that had a significant bearing on the evident differences between river drawings. That may lead to the setting of new goals and strategies to get to a better state of life flow. Others, influenced by differing cultural leanings, may prefer to focus on process and enable a discussion of: 'How things are going for you right now'. Each approach, or a combination of the two, is possible because of the broader contextual view that the Kawa model affords. When the Kawa metaphor is sensitively and respectfully advanced, the therapeutic relationship between client and occupational therapist can be strengthened and used in a positive and constructive way.

Like real rivers in nature, and real life circumstances in the human experience, the client's residual river may not necessarily be rid of all impediments to life flow. Rocks, driftwood and the usual contour and thickness of the Kawa sides and bottom, will probably change (for the better) but may not disappear altogether. Some problems remain – some social and physical environmental (rocks) factors may have been decreased in size and altered in placement, and remain as a residual in the client's existing river. Some of the client's personality traits (driftwood) may still remain, unaltered or unchanged.

Who Draws, Who Interprets?

In the spirit of the holistic and integrative view of self and nature embodied in the Kawa metaphor, the issue of who actually draws the river diagram is of secondary importance. It may be safe to say that the initial suggestion put forward here is that both client (in the broader sense, which includes collectives) and the occupational therapist produce the diagram. Suffice it to say, the end diagram must be satisfactory to the client, making sure that the narrative of circumstances and context that gives meaning to the client's experience of life is justifiably conveyed through the metaphor. Ensuring that this indeed happens is only possible through an intimate dialogue between therapist and client, where statements and probing questions are intensely used to emerge and clarify an accurate depiction of the client's world view. This is requisite for the process to be truly client-centred and for subsequent therapy to be relevant, meaningful and effective for the client.

Naturally, if the metaphor of the river for life is familiar enough and the client is comfortable expressing themselves through it, then it might be best for the client to proceed with the drawing. The actual drawing of the image can be a valuable point of analysis in itself. Is the client slow and methodical in rendering the image? Does the image look simple, or haphazardly drawn and lacking in any detail? Is there extraordinary detail in the drawing? These characteristics of process might mean something significant in the context of the client's culture, as well as being a gauge for the client's functional performance levels.

Clients and therapists who have been socialised into contexts where individualism and the idea of self-efficacy is familiar and celebrated, may be challenged with the holistic interpretation of the river metaphor. The consciousness of separating the world into distinct entities and into ranked categories is frequently expressed in frustration with the seeming absence of a centrally defined and positioned self. This is a clear cultural limitation of the river metaphor used in this way. Many who hold a more rational view of self and nature will draw their river diagrams and construct the self as a distinct person swimming in the river or even riding in a boat or surfing on top of it. For the Kawa model to be effectively used, the conscious awareness or social construction of 'me *in* the world', as opposed to 'me *against* the world', is favoured.

In some cultures, verbal communication might be preferred over graphic symbols, to convey ideas and feelings. In these cases, the occupational therapist can rely on verbal analogies of the river (or other) metaphors with the same aim – of drawing accurate narratives of the client's experiences in context. The occupational therapist may prefer to take these oral recordings and translate them diagrammatically into a Kawa image.

In some situations, depending on social cultural norms, as we will see in some of the case studies in the next chapter, the occupational therapist may be the one to draw the river. The therapist in these cases will attempt to interpret the client(s)' narratives and derive a river diagram to use as a common metaphor for dialogue. The aim, stated again, is to arrive at a mutual understanding of the client's experience of well-being and disablement and the rich surrounding context that gives these issues their quality and meaning. Ideally the identification, quality and placement of the river components will be determined through a dialogue between all parties involved. The most accurate depiction of the client's context, as the client sees things, will lead to the most meaningful and effective interventions.

Documentation

Although not always explicit, occupational therapists actually use theory in profound and complex ways. Behind every occupational therapist's SOAP (Subjective, Objective, Analysis, Plan) or POR (Problem Oriented (medical) Record) entry is a complex array of thoughts that have filtered through a number of organising frameworks. We may be far from the day when occupational therapists enter river diagrams into the patient medical record charts(!), but the evidence of the Kawa's influence in deriving robust, accurate, meaningful and context laden observations of a client's occupational state of being is certainly apparent. We continue to practise within the cultures of medicine, institutions and health professions that come with their own respective sets of procedures and regulations or norms and these entities structure and influence how occupational therapists document their activities. The Kawa model can take its place among occupational therapy frameworks from which occupational therapists can choose as a means by which occupational therapy goals, practice and evaluation are derived and guided. It may serve as a powerful organising framework to the therapist's reports of the client's progress, as well as in decisions regarding occupational therapy intervention and discharge from care.

How Does *Your* River Flow?

In order to get a sense of whether the Kawa model is relevant to your cultural situation and needs, take a few minutes to try the model on your own situation. If you are an occupational therapy educator, you may want to trial the model on your students, asking them to practise by trialling the model on one another. The ensuing discussion on the Kawa model and the use of theory in occupational therapy is a potentially rich educational experience that invariably follows. The case study contributed by A. Nelson, in the following chapter, is an example of how the Kawa framework can be applied in an educational setting.

On a blank piece of paper, draw a picture of a river meandering out of the distant mountains to your present location, at a self-determined point of the river as it flows towards the sea. Along the river's course, think back in time, reminisce and write some notes about events that occurred that had a significant bearing on shaping and regulating the strength of flow in your life. You may want to use a large piece of paper!

Now let's concentrate on the 'here and now'. Draw a large cross-section of your life's river at this present time and go through the various components of the Kawa as outlined in the previous chapter. You may want to also take another look at the first three stages of implementation contained in this chapter, while mapping out your river.

So, what does your social environment look like? Does it constrain or enable flow by exerting its influence on the shape and channel volume at this point in your river? What kinds of rocks do you have? How many do you have and what are their relative sizes? Where in the river image do these rocks fit? What is the meaning of their interface with elements of the social and physical environment? Do they rest against certain entities in the environment, and/or against other rocks and structures?

What are your driftwood and do they potentially enable or hamper your life flow in those areas?

Where is your water flowing strongest and where are the gaps between structures where life is flowing at a trickle?

You may notice that in this view, everything in your life is part of the same frame. Changing one part of it changes the whole in some way. As the magnitude of one component increases or decreases, the relative magnitude and relationship with all other structures in the same frame will change.

If you could perform occupational therapy on yourself, then where would you focus it and what are some strategies to make it happen? You may want to develop a table of your own 'Kawa Occupational Issues', with an adjoining column to record notes about what you plan to do about these issues, to enable stronger life flow. Some of this is fun and some of this can represent a real challenge. If life were simple and easy, there would not be much need for occupational therapy. The sensation of performing this Kawa exercise is not unlike what it may be like for your clients using the model. Some of these deeply personal and private matters may remain suppressed and hidden, until the proper season comes along to reveal parts of them. At times, they may remain as simple diagrammatic figures that cannot be readily named. It is alright to turn your attention to those other channels of life flow that are ready for attention. Everything has its time, everything has its season. Let nature take its course. Not everything has to be dealt with in a rational straight path through the issue. At least, that is an Eastern way.

Understanding and appreciating the client in context of his or her cultural frame is one of the main mandates in the use of the Kawa model. Until now, occupational therapists have taken some pride in touting a 'client-centred' approach as being one of occupational therapy's hallmarks. Yet, we have a tendency to contradict this basic value in how we construct and put our theoretical materials into practice. Taking any narrative of human occupation that favours a particular slice of Western life, infused with certain culturally bound ideals, social norms and world views into other cultural settings and then proclaiming its universal effectiveness and appropriateness is but a sorely misguided illusion. We may claim our methods to be culturally safe[8] and client centred but in the end, when our client narratives are translated back into the lexicon, concepts and explanatory structures of our universal models, something substantial is lost.

The Kawa model, properly used in clinical settings, should function to provide a broader picture of the person's occupational state beyond and consequent to the medically defined reason that brought the client into occupational therapy. A broader picture enables a broader, more meaningful, occupational therapy. Meeting people where they are at in their life courses, and enabling them to maximise their life flow in a culturally meaningful, relevant and powerfully effective way, is the essence to this occupational therapy.

REFERENCES

[1] Glaser BG. Theoretical Sensitivity. Mill Valley: Sociology Press; 1978

[2] Ellen RF. The cognitive geometry of nature: a contextual approach. In: Descola P, Pálsson G (eds), Nature and Society: Anthropological Perspectives. London: Routledge; 1996; 103–123

[3] Ingold T. The Perception of the Environment: Essays on Livelihood, Dwelling and Skill. London: Routledge; 2000

[4] Ehrmann M. Desiderata. Los Angeles: Brooke House; 1972

[5] Iwama M. The issue is … toward culturally relevant epistemologies in occupational therapy. American Journal of Occupational Therapy 2003; 57(5):582–588

[6] Law M, Baptiste S, Carswell A, McColl M, Polatajko H, Pollock N. Canadian Occupational Performance Measure, 2nd edn. Toronto: CAOT Publications; 1994

[7] Kielhofner GA. Model of Human Occupation: Theory and Application, 3rd edn. Baltimore: Williams and Wilkins; 2002

[8] Ramsden I. *Kawa whakaruruhau* – cultural safety in nursing education in Aotearoa: report to the Ministry of Education. Wellington: Ministry of Education; 1990

Rivers in Context

Brief Narratives and Cases Demonstrating Uses of the
Kawa Model

流

流

Rosemary Hagedorn[1] stressed the importance for occupational therapists to be educated in learning how to think as opposed to being told what to think or what to do[2]. In order for conceptual models of practice to support the acquisition of this essential skill, occupational therapists require frameworks and tools that provide the guidance and means to mine and illuminate client issues in an appropriate context, rather than frameworks that impose a particular set of interests, values, social norms and provide or presuppose *the answers*.

The Kawa model encourages exploration, debate and discussion and does not force a fixed and predominant view or way of understanding the client's situation. Each client and occupational therapist is unique and the contexts that inform and give shape to their uniqueness are to be explored and celebrated. Ultimately, the model seeks to return power to the client by giving credence to their occupational life and issues in the context of the client's perspective of reality rather than imposing a prescribed framework of concepts and principles raised out of another experiential context of experience.

Eight diverse narratives and cases demonstrating culturally relevant applications of the Kawa model set in a variety of international settings are presented in this chapter. The narratives and cases are relatively brief but they should give the reader a sense of the diversity, depth and breadth of the possibilities of the Kawa model. A particular position or vantage repeated throughout this book is about the valid existence of diverse world views, varying constructions of reality and the cultural contexts that inform these respectively. No one model or conceptual framework can adequately validate and translate such diversities in patterns and meanings of daily life.

Likewise, readers may notice that there is not one standard way for interpreting and applying the Kawa model, nor any proprietary instruments and tests wedded to it. Culture and world views are not just the domain of client embodiment but they also affect the occupational therapist and the social frame in which occupational therapy practice unfolds. These cases demonstrate the cultural situatedness of the occupational therapist and his or her occupational therapy. Readers will come to understand their own cultural situation and culture bound views of reality and truth while considering these diverse cases. This may be experienced as uneasiness and even perhaps in some sense of dissonance with the processes being explained. That dissonance may be experienced and witnessed in comments like: 'Oh, I don't understand why that therapist decided to do that'; 'I would have never arrived at that conclusion'; 'uh-oh, the client missed the real problem altogether!'

In these responses resides an essential cultural lesson of the Kawa model. Truth is relevant to cultural situation, and the truths we think we see in making sense of our clients' occupational worlds are informed by a unique context of experiences and acquired knowledge that, in all probability, will differ (even if only slightly) from the very contexts of experience and acquired knowledge of our own. To welcome and embrace the emergence of the clients' truths, and to accord them power by fashioning occupational therapy accordingly in meaningful and truly enabling ways, is the essence of culturally relevant occupational therapy.

The Kawa model provides occupational therapists with an alternative way to understand the day-to-day occupational experiences of their patients and clients in context. The model is not a universal framework into which clients must translate or fit their views of reality. There are no preconstructed concepts into which the client must allow an occupational therapist to bend or force their occupational narratives. Rather, the Kawa model is meant to be a malleable vehicle that the client can exploit for the purpose of bringing their precious narratives into the potentially enabling realm of occupational therapy. Fitting the mandate of occupational therapy to the client's requirements, rather than requiring the client to fit the mandate of occupational therapy, represents a challenging way of thinking in this contemporary profession. In this way, the Kawa model represents a revolutionary development in the comprehension and use of theoretical material in occupational therapy. The model is but one example of the kind of client- and culture-relevant theoretical frameworks that occupational therapists may need to develop in order to move their practice in a more equitable, inclusive and meaningful direction.

Each of the contributions in the following pages, given by occupational therapists with extensive practice experience, is brief and does not follow a uniform format. Several of these cases, particularly those from Japan, were translated into English. In keeping with the theme of cultural relativity, these vignettes remain culturally situated. They are presented 'as is' for the reader to consider from his or her own contexts of experience and world views, and to imagine how the Kawa metaphor and its associated concepts might relate to their own culturally situated practice contexts. Therefore, readers are encouraged to examine these cases with a critical eye, and consider how the Kawa model might be modified to fit the requirements of the occupational therapist's and client's particular cultural contexts.

The Kawa Model As a Window into Client Occupational Contexts: The Case of Pedro Mendez

Michael Iwama BSc, BScOT, MSc, PhD, OT(c)

Associate Professor, Department of Occupational Science & Occupational Therapy

University of Toronto, Toronto, Canada

Mr Pedro Mendez has been referred to an outpatient rehabilitation programme by his physician. He is 66 years old and had come to live with his son's family in this North-Eastern city almost 4 years ago from Central

America. Spanish is Mr Mendez's native language but he speaks English well enough for normal conversations.

Mr Mendez has been diagnosed with osteoarthritis and his chart reads that he needs some help with his ability to perform his self-care and activities of daily living (ADL) tasks. X-ray scans have indicated that the osteoarthritis affects Mr Mendez's lumbar spine and right hip. Despite all of your efforts to elicit information from him regarding his meaningful occupations, treatment planning (i.e. goals) to restore his independence in daily living activities, he seems despondent and at times evasive.

He does not participate in any of the therapeutic group activities, preferring to stay on the periphery. He is not overtly disruptive and usually does what he is asked to do in terms of therapy. When Mr Mendez is asked about his hobbies and usual routines at home, he defers to his family members to speak for him. 'Please ask my son when he comes for me.' In rounds, the team discusses his case and after 2 weeks of the same pattern, comes to the conclusion that he is being 'non-compliant' in a 'passive-aggressive' kind of way. 'He's just going through the motions … he doesn't want to be here, so let him finish this week of treatment and discharge him!' your colleagues aver, speaking from a feeling of frustration. 'We've tried our best. It can't be helped; it's his culture.'

The occupational therapist committed to an occupation-based view of the client, decides to go beyond the usual rehabilitation service protocols and tries an alternate approach based on a framework geared towards understanding the client's occupational life in a broader context. The Kawa model, a new framework developed outside of the Western hemisphere, is tried.

Using the River metaphor as a framework to understand more profoundly the contextual nature of Mr Mendez's difficulties and challenges from his perspective, the occupational therapist begins to raise and appreciate the multi-faceted and complex dimensions of his experience of life in the present.

Mr Mendez's Kawa

The occupational therapist finds that Mr Mendez and his family are part of a small, closely knit ethnic community of Guatemalan immigrants. He and his family are careful not to make any trouble, nor bring any shame on the community. His care and health-seeking behaviour is constrained by the regulations of his health insurance policies and other factors. More than his back pain, which was the reason listed for his referrals, he reveals he is worried about his family situation. His son is apparently having difficulties with his work permit and is resisting deportation. And under these conditions Mr Mendez reports that 'everything hurts'.

He complains of his nagging back pain: 'everything I do hurts … I am afraid to make it worse'. 'I am afraid that I cannot perform the usual functions of a man – I can't even embrace my grandchildren'. 'I feel worthless, I cannot help around the house and I have become a burden to my family. I have lost confidence in my abilities.' Mr Mendez is often heard whispering to his wife, who passed away a year ago. When asked about whom he is speaking with, tears well up in his eyes while he replies – 'Oh, I miss her so terribly; I talk with her all the time'.

'If I can get better, the first thing I want to do is play with my grandchildren, and of course, take my dog to the park twice a day.'

The therapist sits down with Mr Mendez and his life situation, past and present, is talked about through the River metaphor. A therapeutic relationship of trust begins to form as the therapist listens to the client and verifies the symbolic meaning of the river drawing and its emerging components.

Mr Mendez's river (life force) is flowing weakly. The impedance to flow is due to a complex collection of numerous factors (such as physical, social, political, medical, financial) that are interconnected. Figure 9.1 portrays Mr Mendez's river. An inventory of Pedro Mendez's occupational issues are categorised in Table 9.1.

Some may argue that problems like 'the fear of deportation', which has political and socio-economic relevance, is not an occupational therapy issue. From the viewpoint of the Kawa framework, occupation is inextricably tied to matters of life, and any contextual factor that impacts on or influences the form, function and meaning of occupations, qualifies as an occupational therapy interest. The

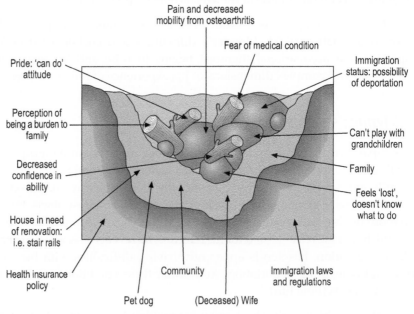

Figure 9.1 Cross-sectional view of Mr Mendez's river, summarising important aspects of his occupational context.

TABLE 9.1 INVENTORY OF PEDRO MENDEZ'S OCCUPATIONAL ISSUES CATEGORISED ACCORDING TO KAWA MODEL CONCEPTS

Kawa concept	Definition	Client-centred issues
Rocks	Discrete circumstances that are considered to impede one's water or *life flow*. They are life circumstances perceived by the client to be problematic and difficult to remove	Pain and decreased mobility from osteoarthritis Immigration status: possibility of deportation Can't play with grandchildren Can't fulfill family duties Feels 'lost', doesn't know what to do
River walls and bottom	The client's environment, in the context of being inseparable from all of the other river structures – namely water and rocks	**Micro level:** Family House – stairs without rails (Deceased) Wife Community Pet dog 'Toro' **Macro level:** Health insurance policy Immigration laws and regulations
Driftwood	The client's personal attributes and resources that can positively or negatively affect the subject's circumstance and life flow. They are transient in nature	Fear of medical condition Pride, 'can do' attitude Perception of being a burden to family Decreased confidence in ability
Water	The subject's *life energy* or *life flow*	Water continues to flow in substantial volume around his arthritis and functional consequences, driftwood (see cell above), and his social and physical environment. Water still flows, but to a lesser extent, through seams and gaps bounded by the structures and components in Mr Mendez's river diagram
Spaces and gaps	Occupational therapy	Potential occupational therapy treatment approaches and points of interventions are in the gaps and channels through which water (life energy) still courses (see Water cell above) and the specific structures that form the boundaries

beauty, power and promise of occupational therapy have always resided in its holistic regard for the client, appreciated in context. The intervention may involve or even be carried out by other health professionals but the relation between these factors and a client's occupations are nonetheless monitored.

Using the river framework to explicate the complex context of Mr Mendez's circumstances, the OT begins to identify those channels where Mr Mendez's life (water) continues to flow. These channels are bounded by his existing problems and challenges (rocks), residual abilities and liabilities (driftwood), and aspects of his physical and social environment (river walls and sides). Intervention is, like his circumstances, multi-faceted, involving a combination of foci and approaches. Rocks might be eroded through a variety of approaches and interventions, including the use of purposeful activity and education. For example, the river walls and bottom might be expanded through family and client discussions to facilitate greater understanding and support for Mr Mendez. Modifications to his home environment might be targeted to enable greater ability and safety. A social worker and psychologist may be brought in for delicate matters requiring categorisation. Advocacy for Mr Mendez's family in accessing legal counsel for immigration issues maybe in order. Possible occupational therapy interventions for Pedro Mendez's occupational issues, categorised according to Kawa model concepts are listed in Table 9.2.

As the river contents and structure expand, the channels become wider and the client's life force is liberated to flow more strongly and fully. The essence of occupational therapy from this regard is to enhance or enable greater life flow. If matters of occupation are supposed to be at the centre of occupational therapy, then its approaches ought to be comprehensive, contextual and client centred. As more information emerges about the characteristics of Mr Mendez's river, the intervention becomes more profound and focused (Figure 9.2).

A Japanese Interpretation and Application of the Kawa Model in a Context of Mental Health Practice

Naoe Yoshimura OTR

Staff Occupational Therapist

Makibi Hospital, Kurashiki, Japan

Hiroko Fujimoto MscOT, OTR (then of Asahigawa Jidouin Hospital for Children) aided in the translation and preparation of the author's Japanese manuscript into English. Currently, Ms Fujimoto is affiliated with the Makibi Hospital in Okayama, Japan, and Aino University, Osaka, Japan

Reconciling conventional occupational therapy conceptual models, which emphasise independence and self-determinism, among a host of concepts emerged from Western cultural contexts, to Japanese constructions of reality that are intertwined with collective social values, represents a fundamental

Kawa concept	Client-centred issues	Occupational therapy actions
	TABLE 9.2 POSSIBLE OCCUPATIONAL THERAPY INTERVENTIONS FOR PEDRO MENDEZ'S OCCUPATIONAL ISSUES, CATEGORISED ACCORDING TO KAWA MODEL CONCEPTS	
Rocks	Pain and decreased mobility from osteoarthritis Immigration status: possibility of deportation Can't play with grandchildren Can't fulfill family duties Feels 'lost', doesn't know what to do	Attend arthritis activity group. Exercise and education on body mechanics. Joint preservation approaches and techniques. Social work consult for Mr Mendez (and family) to discuss immigration situation. Problem solve to look at possible activities that Mr Mendez can share with his grandchildren. Coordinate with other team members, such as nursing, psychology, social work to set up a series of family conferences to discuss role and family duties, ways to give Mr Mendez more avenues to find a way though his disability experience
River walls and bottom	**Micro level:** Family House – stairs without rails (Deceased) Wife Community Pet dog 'Toro' **Macro level:** Health insurance policy Immigration laws and regulations	Coordinate with psychologist or social worker to address possible issues of concern through family conferences: particularly in regard to roles and expectations. Acknowledge Mr Mendez's loss of life partner as profoundly important and qualify his ongoing relationship with his wife as a legitimate and meaningful occupation. Examine ways and means to keep Mr Mendez involved in his community, including support he may need. Work to enable his occupations around his relationship of his dog. Home visit with aim to assess his residence to make it safe and enabling given his condition. Refer Mr Mendez to social work to examine health insurance policy (in strict confidence). Ask Social Worker to look at resources in the community to gain credible information regarding immigration, and immigration counselling
Driftwood	Fear of medical condition Pride, 'can do' attitude Perception of being a burden to family Decreased confidence in ability	Provide pertinent information; use Spanish interpreter or materials, regarding his medical condition. Coordinate with psychologist or social worker to address possible issues of guilt and worry through family conferences. Utilise graded mastery types of activity formats to provide Mr Mendez with feedback on his progress

185

Table continued over…

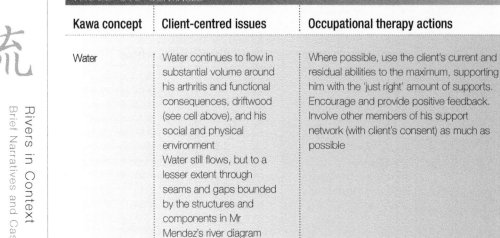

TABLE 9.2 CONTINUED

Kawa concept	Client-centred issues	Occupational therapy actions
Water	Water continues to flow in substantial volume around his arthritis and functional consequences, driftwood (see cell above), and his social and physical environment Water still flows, but to a lesser extent through seams and gaps bounded by the structures and components in Mr Mendez's river diagram	Where possible, use the client's current and residual abilities to the maximum, supporting him with the 'just right' amount of supports. Encourage and provide positive feedback. Involve other members of his support network (with client's consent) as much as possible

challenge in Japanese occupational therapy practice. In a collective society where 'belonging' is strongly tied to experiences of 'being' and self-identity, those who cannot demonstrate adequate social ability are susceptible to stigma and denied membership and participation in mainstream Japanese society. The stigma is collective and implicates family, social networks, community and the work place. A new model of occupational therapy recently

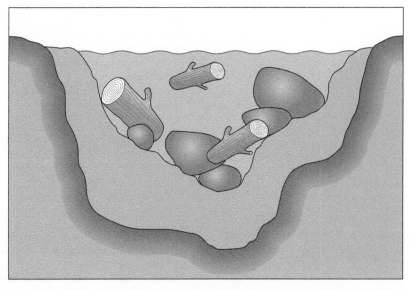

Figure 9.2 A more comprehensive and multi-faceted occupational therapy approach to Mr Mendez's situation has resulted in stronger life flow. Note that all impediments to flow have not been totally eliminated. Many of the structures have reduced in size and shape, contributing to better flow. Like most people's lives, some struggles and challenges remain and are part of most life experiences.

emerged from the clinical field shows promise in helping to understand the complexities of the experience of mental illness in the Japanese cultural context. Application of the River model will be demonstrated using an example of a mental health client's short stay leave, family adjustment and other challenges implicated by relatively long admissions (spanning decades in certain cases) common in Japanese psychiatric hospitals.

Introduction

The occupational therapy I learned at school was based on the medical model that sees and treats clients accordingly. But my clinical experience gradually made me aware of the limitations of the medical model and the necessity of a more comprehensive model that encompasses both the client and the environment. The Western occupational therapy models that focus on the relationship between human being, occupation and environment are well-known, but the difference in culture makes them difficult to use in Japanese clinical practice.

The Kawa model, or the river model, is something that emerged from discussions among Japanese occupational therapists who shared similar concerns. In this short case presentation I will talk about a case in which the Kawa model was used effectively to represent a client's world as the client constructs it, and to work out a rehabilitation plan for his return to life back in the community.

Japanese Culture

Let me first explain a few characteristics of Japanese culture that surround and strongly affect clients' lives in Japan.

In the West, the individual and environment are treated rationally and perceived as clearly distinguished entities.

In Japan, a human being is considered to be part of the environment and the two cannot exist separately. What is important for most Japanese is a sense of oneness with the environment and harmony with others. Japanese sense of autonomy and identity is unique in that it is closely related to *belonging* to a socially recognised place and ability to exercise appropriate conduct there. The meanings of self-determination and behaviour tend to fluctuate according to the circumstance – according to 'ba' as Japanese people might refer to it.

The Japanese harmonious view of nature is well known; nature is not something we have to confront, nor seek to control. The Japanese relationship between individual and society is similar to that relationship. Japanese clients live in this kind of cultural context.

The Reality of Being Diagnosed As Mentally Ill in Japan

Psychiatric treatment in Japan has a long history of secluded internment with the emphasis on protecting the interests of safety and harmony of society. The majority of Japanese people tend to think that people with mental illness are frightening and uncontrollable, and therefore try to avoid them. Clients and their families, fearful of the social prejudice and discrimination, tend to focus solely on the quick elimination of disorder by medicine, removing the patient from public view, and disregard working on their disability and social handicap.

The following conditions are strongly related to recovery: whether or not clients, as they really are with their existing disability, have a place to belong to, whether or not they have a social relationship in which they can feel safe, and the amount of attention given to enabling the mental health client to harmonise with their circumstances.

The Kawa model is useful to the occupational therapist in understanding the circumstances surrounding a client, including the analyses of the client's belonging, the status of social relationships and other factors affecting the client's state of harmony with the environment.

The River Model and a Case of a Client

Takao is a 49-year-old, single man. He was diagnosed with pseudoneurotic schizophrenia and has been in hospital for the last 3 years. Medical staff would describe Takao as suffering from neurotic symptoms, such as anxiety, depersonalisation, and loss of volition. Extraordinary experiences, as evident in his bizarre behaviour, occur only when he gets very sick. From the time he was diagnosed at age 17, Takao has been in and out of hospital. An overview of Takao's experience with mental illness is represented in Figure 9.3.

Readers of this case situated outside Japan may be shocked by the length of Takao's stay, but Takao doesn't think of it negatively. 'I felt safe in the hospital. I was with people with the same illness and I had someone I could talk to when anxiety attacked me. It was fun to go out for a walk, watch a movie, have coffee and so on, carrying with me such an atmosphere and human relationships. On the other hand, living with my family put a lot of stress on me as I couldn't keep pace with my healthy mother and brother'.

The Kawa model that compares one's life history to a river starting in a mountain and ending in the sea also facilitates a diachronic view of life. The model covers the interrelationships between a client and his environment by using a three-dimensional view of the river, which makes it easier to see one's life in a more comprehensive and positive way. Proper understanding of the changes in clients' environments is crucial to anticipate and respond to the changes of clients themselves who are bound to be affected by the former.

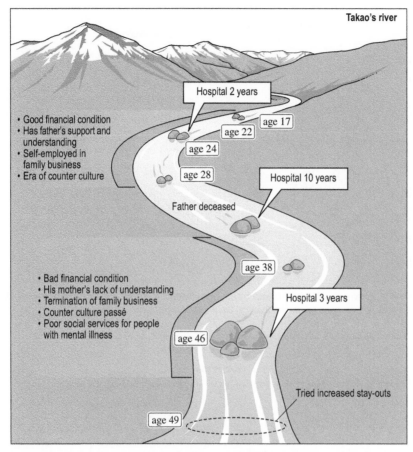

Figure 9.3 Overview of Takao's case as shown through the Kawa image.

We tried to increase Takao's home visit/return to life back in the community, but it didn't work. He was now at home and I asked him how he was doing there. He answered: 'I don't know what to do at home. I feel pressured by my surroundings and I get anxious'. Takao attributed this to his illness. His mother thought the same.

I used the Kawa model and visualised his situation, especially the relationship between him and his environment, as I saw it.

Figure 9.4 is a picture of Takao's river diagram in hospital from his occupational therapist's view.

Figure 9.5 is a picture of Takao's river at home from his occupational therapist's view.

I showed him these river diagram pictures and told him that the difference in environment seems to be one of the reasons why he might be feeling uneasy at home. (In a hierarchically structured society like Japan, the occupational therapist may feel comfortable drawing the Kawa diagram for the client.)

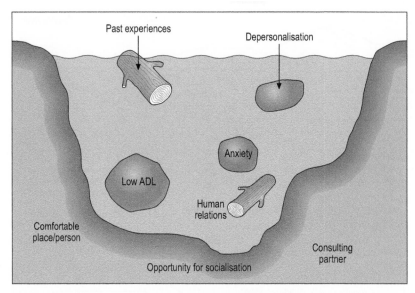

Figure 9.4 Takao's river diagram drawn by the occupational therapist during Takao's hospital stay. Overview of Takao's case as shown through the Kawa image.

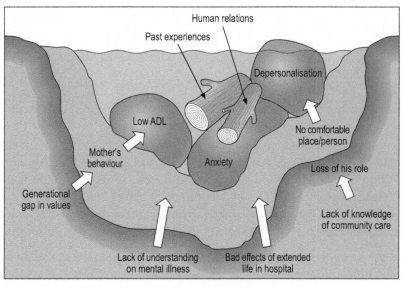

Figure 9.5 Image of Takao's river at home from his occupational therapist's view.

I proposed that we try to create, within the community and using various community care services, an environment not much different from that in the hospital. I also proposed that we talk with his family for understanding and support for our plan.

Takao, told me that the second diagram (Figure 9.5) properly showed his situation at home, but that the first diagram (Figure 9.4) was not right.

So, I asked him to draw a picture of himself in hospital.

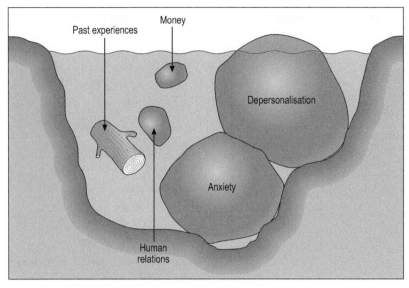

Figure 9.6 Picture of Takao's river adapted from what he drew.

Figure 9.6 is a picture of Takao's river adapted from what he drew.

You can see the difference between Takao's diagram and the first diagram (Figure 9.4) that I drew.

The difference in size of rocks and driftwood and difference in amount of water vividly revealed the gap in our perceptions. Although we were using the same terms, such as *anxiety* and *depersonalisation*, the way he felt and experienced them was different from what I had expected.

It was also made clear that he saw his life as being much more fragile than the way I saw it. I admitted this difference to him. He seemed a little relieved and said: 'You finally have understood my anxiety, haven't you?' He then agreed to have a family meeting.

However, Takao was still feeling anxious about the coming change in his life. I used the Kawa model again to have him reflect on how he coped with his circumstances over the last 3 years. During that span, he somehow managed the changes in environment between hospital and home. My aim was to enable him to feel more secure and more confident in himself. This time I didn't show any Kawa diagrams and just asked him to draw rivers of himself at the time of hospitalisation, at present in hospital, and during occupational therapy sessions (Figure 9.7).

As he was drawing, he talked about how he was feeling in each occasion. He actually realised his recovery and took a positive view of the river. Instead of attributing all the anxieties to his illness, he realised that anxieties necessarily arose from life and that he could get rid of or come to terms with them if he properly faced them. He now agreed to have a community care service

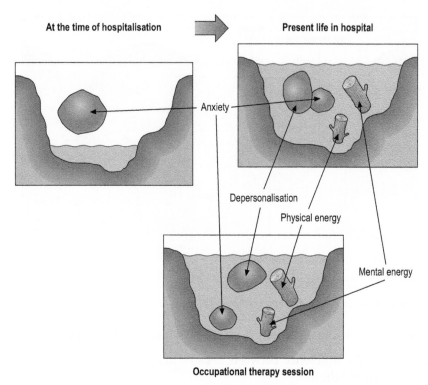

Figure 9.7 River diagrams drawn by Takao, summarising his situation over time.

package developed for him. He also put into language, for the first time, the significance of the occupational therapy he received since it was started.

Occupation in Takao's context was his *life flow*. Occupational therapy carried the potential to enable and maximise that flow.

Like a River, Collective Harmony over Independence in Japanese Occupational Therapy for Children

Hiroko Fujimoto BA, MscOT, OTR

Staff Occupational Therapist

Asahigawa Jidouin Hospital for Children, Okayama, Japan

(Author's affiliation at the time of preparing this vignette. Ms Fujimoto is currently affiliated with the Makibi Hospital in Okayama, Japan and Aino University Osaka, Japan)

Overview

When occupational therapists encounter early childhood clients, it is essential to also know the caregiver's attitudes towards parenting. We need to know what is being expected of the child as she grows, as her world expands and her capabilities change. The life of a 5-year old girl with cerebral palsy is presented using the Kawa model. With this new model the therapist's aim, discussions with the parent, treatment strategies and results can be understood chronologically. The model illustrates that the child's life is shaped by the caregiver's point of view and actions, which are reflexively influenced by the socio-cultural background. The model illuminates the complexities of influential factors and captures the characteristics of Japanese people that give primacy to social harmony over independence. The new model exposes the particular construction of relationships between individuals and their environments in our culture, which previous occupational therapy models could not adequately explain.

The Kawa Model

The metaphor of a river categorises life and flow of events that typify experiences of well-being and difficulty. The river metaphor is composed of water itself and the structures around it, including objects flowing with it and objects that could potentially impede it. The water, flowing in direction, symbolises life itself, spirit and the motivation to live. The water flow is shaped and bounded by the river walls and floor, foliage near the water's edge and by rocks of various sizes. Foliage symbolises human resources around the client, the floor symbolises the family environment and the walls symbolise the social environment. Flotsam, such as driftwood, leaves, refuse, etc., symbolise the client's life history, including sense of values, clinical history and economic situation. At times, these items can obstruct water flow, yet in another instance, can help dislodge, or push through other factors that impede flow. The most significant impediment to flow of life is rocks of various sizes, which represent life circumstances. Rocks may symbolise accidents, illnesses, and other largely unforeseen events. Whenever the flow of water is impeded, occupational therapy is prescribed to restore and maximise the flow. To enhance flow, occupational therapists search for every conceivable advantage, symbolised by cracks or weak points in the rocks and focus the water strength on these points. Breaking through weak points between the rocks and the river walls or floor are also viable strategies. On the whole, occupational therapists try to facilitate the power of water itself to facilitate nature's course.

Case: Naomi

5 years old, female

Medical diagnosis: cerebral palsy (diplegia)

Family: father, mother, sister (9)

Physical therapy since 13 months

Occupational therapy since 21 months

Naomi is a cheerful girl. She likes to play simple games, like 'house' with adults and her sister. Though her hand skills do not let her play as she wants to, when she is interested enough, she plays a lot with toys that require fine motor activities. She can crawl and control her wheelchair for transportation. Her communicative understanding is age-appropriate and she articulates without problems. She understands concepts of numbers, shape, size and colour. She started to go to nursery school in her community at age 3. She spends more time with new groups of people now, expanding her social environment beyond her family.

Refer to Figure 9.8 (1)

The family's expectation for Naomi is for her to walk on her own, to clear the developmental milestones for her age.

The River Appearance

Mother cannot understand the child's needs, making the river floor narrow.

Mother

Concerned with her child not being able to sit or stand. She seems to be more interested in correcting her child's postural alignment than playing with her.

Child

Cannot show her desires and demands. She experiences difficulty in using her hands. Play is often obstructed and she spends time doing nothing or appears unsettled.

OT Goal

To have fun playing and completing each play activity. To get the mother absorbed in play with her daughter.

Refer to Figure 9.8 (2)

The River Appearance

The floor of the river is widened because the mother has started to pay attention to the child's needs.

Mother

Talks often about toys that the child is not able to play with well.

Child

Not interested in being independent in self-care.

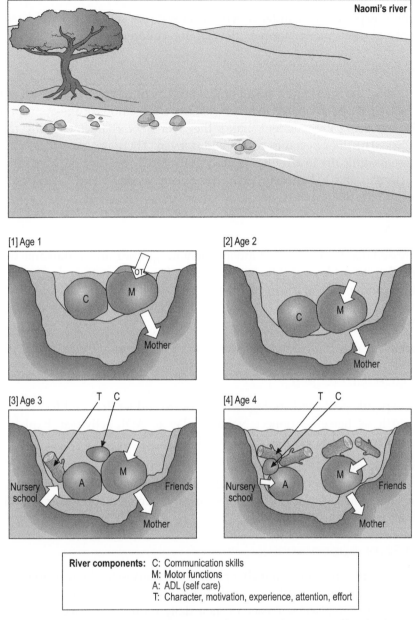

Figure 9.8 Cross-sectional representations of Naomi's river at various stages of her development.

OT Goal/Strategies

Guide the mother to have a more specific goal that corresponds with the child's abilities. The occupational therapist gathers information about her favourite play at home and recommends home programmes.

Refer to Figure 9.8 (3)
Naomi is expected to be independent in her self-care activities. Starts nursery school and meets many 'normal' (developing) children.

The River Appearance

The floor of the river is now greatly influenced by nursery school as well as by her mother. Being compared to other children, expectations of age-appropriate tasks and being independent makes the river floor characteristically more complex. The floor becomes rough and uneven. There is a new rock, which represents difficulty in activities of daily living (ADL) acquisition. Motivations for activities and her cheerful character appear as driftwood, acting on the rocks and the floor of the river.

Mother

Depressed that her child is not independent in self-care, and at the same time, wants her to achieve it. She watches over her child within the group of children with positive, warm attitude.

Child

Expands her play. She exhibits an increase in attitude towards self-care activities.

OT Goal/Strategies

To set specific goals and strategies for self-care and let the child feel that she can do it by herself. Connect Naomi's play to ADL activities. Explain to Naomi's mother and ask for her cooperation.

Refer to Figure 9.8 (4)
Naomi's mother expects her to be able to share in play with her friends and be independent in self-care, but Naomi's slower movement and lower cognitive abilities frustrate such ambitions.

The River Appearance

Though there is no significant change in the nursery-school (river floor), and because the mother is working to help Naomi by altering the respective environmental factors/issues in each of their daily routines, the overall environment (river floor) is widened. The development of Naomi's motor abilities is represented by a smaller rock. These changes coincide with greater flow.

Mother

Talks about her child cheerfully. In spite of her anxieties to the new environment, she seems happier with her child's development and appears to enjoy child-rearing. She is more optimistic and has a better appreciation for each of her child's daily activities.

Child

Makes her own decisions and lives actively. Naomi expands her interests and her potential for independence is illuminated.

OT Goal/Strategies

Naomi's preparation for primary school. Help Naomi's mother to prepare for changes in the new environment (primary school).

Some Conclusions

* The river shape is influenced by the mother/caregiver's approaches and values

* The river shape is influenced by the changes in the person's social environment, expanding and contracting the river's floor and banks

* What is expected of the person by the caregiver and the society changes according to age. The norms of age-appropriateness are related to the social and cultural context

* By using the Kawa (River) model, we can visualise the chronological changes of the person

* The Kawa model can not only show the approaches for the accomplishment of quantifiable goals, but also can show the surrounding social collective's aims in supporting the client

* The Kawa model helps us to imagine the relationships of occupational therapists to people surrounding the client and make necessary strategies with them

* The Kawa model explicates enabling and disabling factors with regard to the client's flow through the proportional sizes of the river components. These are determined in collaboration with the client(s).

The Kawa Model in Mental Health Contexts: Two Cases from the UK

Kee Hean Lim MSc DipOT PGCEd

Lecturer in Occupational Therapy

Brunel University, Middlesex, UK

I first encountered the Kawa 'River' model while attending the 3rd Asia Pacific Occupational Therapy Congress in Singapore in September 2003. What initially struck me about the Kawa 'River' model, were five key factors. First, its uniqueness as the first ever occupational therapy model to be developed in the

East. Secondly, that the Kawa model arose out of the discourse and limitations experienced by occupational therapists working with existing models of practice. Thirdly, that it was developed by a selection of clinicians in practice, rather than contrived within the pillars of academia, by scholars. Fourthly, the Kawa model's key concepts and features are simple and *natural*. Fifthly, the use of a 'River' as the metaphor within the model, which is an image widely associated and understood by many cross culturally.

As I began to discover and learn more about the Kawa 'River' model, I became increasingly intrigued by its clinical utility and applicability beyond its situated Japanese socio-cultural context. In particular, I was keen to examine its potential utility and relevance within the UK context, where I have worked as an occupational therapist and experienced the limitations of existing prescriptive occupational therapy models of practice.

The first step I undertook prior to utilising and applying the Kawa model was to examine the relevance of it key concepts and features, by undertaking an informal inquiry where a selection of students and clinicians within various fields of practice were recruited and questioned about their conceptual understanding of a 'River'. I was able to ascertain whether the image of a 'River', which is the central tenet of the Kawa model was similarly perceived and associated within the UK context as it was in its original Japanese context. Some of the responses from participants included: 'A river has a beginning and an end'; that 'rivers may compose water, sand, rocks, pieces of wood, fishes'; that 'rivers are a source of life, support and survival'; and that 'rivers have direction and flow'. These varied responses were encouraging in that they reinforced my belief that the concept of a river is associated and under-stood by many cross culturally and with most individuals and communities able to relate their life journey and experiences in terms of a personal and unique river that flows through a passage of time.

Having attained the positive results from the inquiry I decided to pilot the use of the model with several individual clients/service users to examine the clinical utility of the Kawa model. Here are case studies of two distinctly different service users whom I have had the opportunity to examine and capture their experience and circumstances utilising the Kawa model. They shall be known here as Cathy and Krishna, who both suffer from mental health difficulties. Presented are brief examinations of their case histories, pictorial representations of their 'Rivers' at a point in time, and how occupational therapy may be used within the framework of the Kawa model to help them to overcome their difficulties.

One of the key qualities of the Kawa model is its refreshing simplicity. My experience of explaining and utilising the Kawa model with several clients/ service users has reinforced my opinion that the metaphor and concept of a 'River' representing or depicting one's life journey is easily identifiable and understood. This is contrary to my previous experience of utilising some existing Western models of practice, which are infused with complex professional terminology, jargon and technical concepts that are rarely understood by many clinicians let alone their clients within the UK and beyond. Indeed, my first experience of utilising the Kawa model with both Cathy and Krishna proved reassuring, as they were almost immediately able to comprehend, understand and relate their life journey in terms of a personal river.

Krishna

Krishna is a 34-year-old male of South Asian ethnicity. He is single and lives with his family. Krishna is very friendly, sociable and spends much of his time using computers, which he enjoys very much. He was diagnosed with schizophrenia and has a 15-year history of mental illness. He has had a history of numerous relapses but is currently compliant with his medication regimen. He has poor concentration and self-care skills.

Krishna is currently receiving long-term sickness benefits. He has an intermittent work history, but is currently keen to do some voluntary work. Krishna is surrounded by a strong and supportive social network of friends and family members. His family is very supportive, although they can appear to be overly concerned at times. Krishna regularly attends his appointments with his occupational therapists and community psychiatric nurse.

With Krishna, I was able to observe him gaining greater awareness and understanding of how his personal river reflected his life journey and how the rocks in his river were symbolic or representative of the difficulties he was experiencing. We were able also to focus on his assets and strengths (driftwood and spaces) in terms of his friendly and sociable disposition, his previous computer skills, his desire to engage in work and examine how we could utilise these positive aspects in overcoming his difficulties. During this process, Krishna identified the rocks within his river as representing his poor concentration, his history of mental illness and periods of relapse. His initial depiction of his river allowed for a process of examination and discussion on what he considered to be his difficulties and what his family and occupational therapist identified as an additional potential rock, i.e. his self-care needs, which he had not previously perceived to be an area of concern (Figure 9.9).

Krishna's Occupational Therapy Intervention Guided by the Kawa Model

Water

The aim of occupational therapy is to maximise Krishna's life flow. This will involve reducing and removing elements that presently impede his river's flow and maximising existing channels or spaces where his water currently flows.

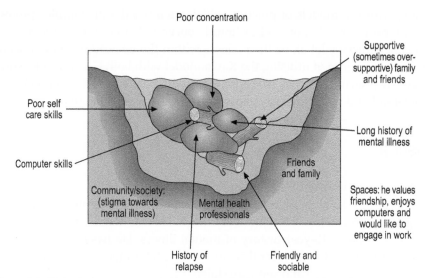

Figure 9.9 Krishna's river as summarised and drawn by the occupational therapist.

Rocks

Identify the rocks, their relative size and location. Determine with Krishna (and his family) which obstacles are most troublesome to him.

Krishna and his family report that he is not able to look after his self-care.

Manipulate the rocks: reduce the obstacles by providing help with self-care skills including personal grooming, laundry and meal preparation. Monitor his mental health status. Work on increasing his concentration skills (through participation in relevant/meaningful activities, such as computer skills training).

Spaces/Channels

Identify current and potential spaces, and their location, paying attention to the context surrounding the flow. Determine which spaces are most important and meaningful to Krishna.

Maximising the spaces: promoting his inner strength, interest, abilities and skills. These may include: work preparation training, exploring voluntary work, attending the local sports centre to meet new friends and build stamina, and working on his personal CV.

River Bed and Sides

Widen the river sides and deepen the river bottom:

• Consult with benefits advisor to assess Krishna's benefit status in relation to paid voluntary work.

- Provide support for Krishna and his family in terms of regular family meetings to help the family understand Krishna's condition and his desire to engage in voluntary work, and to do more for himself.

- Facilitate a process to involve his whole professional team and family in supporting his engagement in voluntary work, his social interests and computer skills training.

Driftwood

Identify aspects of character and attributes, and materials that may act as assets or liabilities in the Krishna's life flow. Determine Krishna's cultural and social context, towards an understanding of factors that will help or hinder his occupational well-being.

Utilise the driftwood: enhance the positive aspects of his character and attributes – friendliness, desire for voluntary work, build on his computer skills etc. Getting his family to support his desire to get fit, socialise and engage in work etc.

The use of the model provided the opportunity to examine how Krishna's perspectives, priorities and concerns were different from those of his family. An additional advantage of the pictorial representation of Krishna's 'River', was its use as a visual catalyst within the family sessions for discussion and debate. Krishna's parents were able to understand some of the issues and concerns that Krishna perceives as hurdles and barriers that restricted him from achieving more and getting better. They were also able to understand how they might be able to assist him in achieving what he wanted in terms of his future goals.

Cathy

Cathy is a 38-year-old, Caucasian woman who has been diagnosed with depression and obsessive compulsive disorder (OCD). Although Cathy has a few close friends, she has virtually no contact with her family. She reportedly had a difficult childhood marked by psychological abuse and being a victim of bullying in school.

Cathy has varied interests which include fashion and clothing, food, especially Indian, and music in which she pays special attention to Abba. Cathy is resilient, having overcome much in her life. She is friendly. In regard to her work skills, she has developed secretarial skills and office clerk experience. Still, she demonstrates poor self-care, hoarding, and low motivation.

Figure 9. 10 depicts Cathy's river as summarised and drawn by the occupational therapist.

Cathy mentioned that undertaking the process of drawing her own river provided her with a real sense of being actively involved in her own treatment.

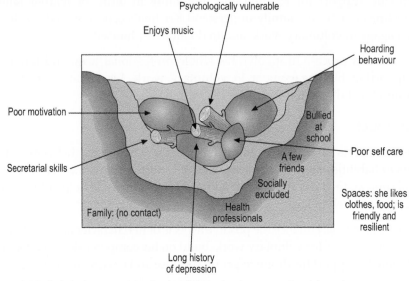

Figure 9.10 Cathy's river as summarised and drawn by the occupational therapist.

She also mentioned that having drawn a collection of cross-sections of her river both from her past, present and future had allowed her to trace her illness journey and helped her gain insight. Highlighting some of the contributing factors that had led her to her present circumstances further helped her to understand what steps she might have to take in order to remain well and to make progress for the future. In Cathy's case, the use of the Kawa model to frame her context, attributes and circumstances, enabled the occupational therapist to draw upon Cathy's resilience and friendly personality as assets to enhance her improvement.

Cathy's Occupational Therapy Intervention Guided by the Kawa Model

Water

The aim of occupational therapy is to maximise Cathy's life flow. This involves reducing and removing elements that impede her river's flow and maximising existing channels or spaces where her water currently flows.

Rocks

Identify the rocks and work with Cathy to reduce these obstacles. Maximising her motivation and self-care through utilising her desire to attend an 'Abba' tribute concert and interest in clothes.

Work on her hoarding behaviour, by means of individual goal-setting sessions to work through organising and clearing her belongings.

Providing psycho-education about depression and OCD.

Spaces/Channels

Identify potential spaces and the context of her river, while determining the areas most important to Cathy.

Maximising spaces through utilising her resilience to explore adult education opportunities in fashion design and cookery.

Maximising the support of close friends to encourage Cathy to socialise more and to take up music classes.

River Bed and Sides

Widen the river sides and deepen the river bed, through determining if Cathy would like to re-establish contact with her family.

Work with Cathy's friends and the MDT (Mental Disabilities Team) to ensure that they aware and support her goal of engaging in adult education and her leisure interest.

Work with the adult education institution and course leaders to ensure support and inclusion for Cathy.

Offer Cathy the opportunity to be referred for psychological help to examine her experience of being bullied at school.

Driftwood

Identify aspects of her character and attributes that may enhance her life flow. Examine Cathy's socio-cultural context to understand factors that may help or hinder her health, recovery and well-being.

Enhance the positive aspects, like Cathy's resilience, friendliness and her interest in music and past secretarial skills.

Engaging with her friends to support her interest and support her health and well-being.

Importantly, although Krishna and Cathy had distinctly diverse ethnic, social and contextual experiences, they were similarly able to apply the concepts held within the Kawa model. Capturing and making sense of their own experiences and gaining insight into how they could influence and bring change to their circumstances were common outcomes from this process.

The Kawa model, I feel, possesses several advantages and qualities over other existing conceptual models. Uniquely, the Kawa model, with its close links to Eastern/holistic philosophy, regards each person as possessing within themselves the human potential or inner spirit to recover and overcome personal circumstances. This is a concept that is neglected within the majority of existing conceptual models. The Kawa model further enables the clinician and client to focus on the holistic interplay of factors such as strengths, difficulties, assets, circumstances, pressures that may have an impact on the individuals' river flow and ultimate health and well-being.

The Kawa model also views the individual within the wider context in which they exist and the impact and influence that the familial, social, environmental, professional, political and economic context may play in supporting or limiting the individual's journey towards health and recovery. Most existing models require the mastery of a series of technical terms, professional jargon and terminology, often understood by few clients and their carers (and even occupational therapists!). The visual qualities of the Kawa model, its naturalistic concepts and simplicity of application, enhances the clients' ability to understand and personally relate the focus of occupational therapy intervention.

Mental health practice in the UK has experienced a positive shift away from paternalism towards concepts of service user empowerment and involvement. The key philosophy and features of the Kawa 'River' model correspond well with these new principles and focus.

Occupational therapists in mental health have long subscribed to the principle of journeying with the client through their illness and health in order to enable recovery. The Kawa model promotes this perspective, enabling both the client and professional to view the application of the Kawa model as a process or journey shared, as both parties examine the flow of the client's river. The Kawa model also supports the concept of client/person focus interventions, requiring the professional to work along the client in constructing and understanding the course of the river flow and the potential for change. The focus on a holistic perspective presented within the model, prompts the professional to pay additional attention on the collective and wider environmental factors that impact on the individual. This supports the focus in the UK of advocating and tackling issues of social exclusion and marginalisation in partnership with and on behalf of the client/service user.

My personal thoughts and experiences of using the Kawa model have been positive. I have found the key concepts and features of the model are equally understood by clinicians, clients and their carers alike. The simplicity of the Kawa model, which is devoid of linear lines, circle and boxes, as represented in many existing occupational therapy models, enhances utility and application for both the clinician and the client. The flexibility of the model, without prescribed and fixed rules in which the model must be practised, allows for greater cross-cultural application and individual adaptation. While most other occupational therapy models are outcome focused, the Kawa model functions as a process model that fosters an exploratory and explanatory examination of the individual contextual perspectives, issues and circumstances. The model promotes the opportunity to explore the narrative/lived experience of the individual, as opposed to predetermined structured and rigid spheres of meaning. The fact that the Kawa model has been developed from the clinical context also resonates well with clinicians who have been introduced to the model here in the UK. The simplicity in utilising the Kawa model and its flexibility and adaptability to being used alongside existing assessments deemed most suitable and appropriate to the individual client, promotes the concept and practice of client/person focused care.

Using a Culturally Relevant Conceptual Model in Japanese Occupational Therapy Clinical Fieldwork Education

Terumi Hatsutori BA OTR

Staff Occupational Therapist

Kawasaki Medical School Hospital, Kurashiki, Japan

Hiroko Fujimoto MscOT, OTR (then of Asahigawa Jidouin Hospital for Children) aided in the translation and preparation of the author's Japanese manuscript into English. Currently, Ms Fujimoto is affiliated with the Makibi Hospital in Okayama, Japan, and Aino University Osaka, Japan

In Japan, OT education is still moderated by the biomedical paradigm, which tends to reduce the patient's needs according to matters of pathology and parts. Although occupational therapy theory and knowledge have been widely imported, they tend to reflect Western experiences and social norms and thus fall short of adequately explaining Japanese experiences of reality and occupation. Occupational therapy approaches involve complex and diverse factors, such as the meaning of activity to a client and the influence of the environs and one's own functional challenges. These all occur within a cultural context. The 'River Model of Japanese Occupational Therapy', recently emerged from the experiences of Japanese clinicians and clients, metaphorically expresses the client's life and occupations. In addition to explaining and guiding culturally relevant occupational therapy interventions, the 'River model' can be employed as an effective teaching tool with OT students, to foster a broader regard for the client in meaningful relation to his or her occupations.

Introduction

The vignette presented in the following pages is a portion of a larger research project that examined how Japanese students understand their occupational therapy practice with existing conceptual models. Specifically, this research examined the effectiveness of the Kawa or River model used with students in fieldwork in Western Japan. To guide this portion of research, the following questions were asked: 'How do Japanese students understand their occupational therapy practice?' and 'How does the Kawa (River) model function in Japanese occupational therapy student fieldwork supervision contexts?'

Problems Regarding Current Conceptual Models Guiding and Influencing Occupational Therapy Education

In Japan, the education of occupational therapists began in 1963 with the help of medical doctors. Since then, occupational therapists have been acknowledged as members of the medical health professions. Therefore, our education has focused on issues of recovery from *impairment* and *disability*, caused by *diseases*.

The International Classification of Impairments, Disabilities & Handicaps[3] (ICIDH) has until recently, been the dominant rehabilitation model. Using this framework, the client's problems are understood along impairments, disabilities, and handicaps in linear structure. In the year 2001, the International Classification of Functioning, Disability & Health[4] (ICF) introduced new concepts, such as functioning and participation, but has yet to take hold in the rehabilitation system. Even now, in the field of medically oriented rehabilitation, the client's needs are to be 'without illness or disabilities'. Likewise, occupational therapy practice is still aimed at trying to find out the cause of a given impairment, and that cause then becomes the object of our interventions. It is therefore understandable that Japanese occupational therapy students are taught to focus on disease and impairment and, consequently, have difficulty understanding the client holistically.

In recent years, conceptual models in occupational therapy built in other countries have been introduced to Japan. I have had difficulties in using these models because the concepts are often not translated into Japanese well enough for us to understand, and the differences in our cultures make it difficult for us to use. For example, Japanese people tend not to say things directly and rationally. Japanese patients often express having no hobbies or self-indulging interests. A lot of clients of occupational therapy are not so eager to be independent and the meanings they put to disabilities can differ broadly.

The students learn these foreign conceptual models in school. However, given their cultural incongruence to Japanese social contexts, they are almost impossible to use – certainly this is more so the case in clinical fieldwork in occupational therapy education.

To be honest, working as an occupational therapist in a medical-oriented field, I have often felt that I could easily forget the viewpoint of seeing the client as a whole. As an occupational therapy educator, however, I felt I needed a way to show and explain the client's assets, as well as the cause for the client's problems to the occupational therapy students I supervised, in a more holistic and effective way.

A group of occupational therapists sharing similar concerns got together and, using naturalistic research methods, emerged a meaningful conceptual model. This later came to be explained by the metaphor of a river: the Kawa model.

Summary of the Kawa model:

- Briefly, 'life' is represented metaphorically as an image of a river (Kawa in Japanese)
- The components of the model correspond to elements of a river in nature
- The past is shown as the upper stream
- The future is shown as the lower stream
- Water flows like the experience of life
- Rocks and debris are like problems and circumstances that can impede the flow of life
- The banks and floor of the river stand for the environment that bounds and shapes the quality of flow.

Using this metaphor, we may proclaim that occupational therapy aims to increase life flow.

Occupational therapy, then, according to this model is any active process by the client that works to increase the flow of water or *life*. This might be achieved through increasing the width and depth of the river, which corresponds to the client's social and physical environment, decreasing the size of rocks, or in other words, decreasing the power or effect of the client's disability, and enabling the client's resources to their maximum.

Using the Kawa Model in Student Fieldwork Supervision

Case: Kenji Kawasaki

Male, 70 years old

Medical diagnosis: C3–4 Spinal cord injury resulting in quadriparesis

1 Standard Protocol Approach

Here is an example of a typical appraisal of the client, by the fieldwork OT student, using the standard (medical rehabilitation) protocols (Table 9.3):

The client's chief complaints were: 'Nothing is going to change, whatever I do' and 'My wish is to die'. Hence the student had difficulty trying to find useful strategies. Students reported experiencing difficulties making sense of the client's varied facial expressions in relation to different settings and surrounding environment.

TABLE 9.3 COMPONENTS AND (BRIEF) CONTENTS OF A TYPICAL OCCUPATIONAL THERAPY ASSESSMENT PROTOCOL EMPLOYED BY JAPANESE OCCUPATIONAL THERAPY STUDENTS IN A REHABILITATION SETTING	
Interview	Chief complaint, hobby, history of present illness, etc.
OT evaluation	Vital check, sensory test, MMT, DTR, muscle tone, ROM-T, mental function, ADL-T, etc.
OT problems	ICIDH, inventory of client's assets
Goal	Long-term goal, short-term goal
Programme	A selection of standard SCI occupational therapy activities

MMT, manual muscle testing; DTR, dexterity training; ROM-T, range of motion test; ADL-T, activities of daily living test; SCI, spinal cord injury.

2 The Kawa Model Approach

Using the Kawa model, the student was able to understand clearly that her conventional occupational therapy approach was focused on medically defined impairments and disabilities and not on the inner perspectives of the client. The student was able to imagine what it was that the occupational therapist needed to approach to help the client. She had not integrated and interpreted the information, but the Kawa model framework made it feasible for her to understand the future environment and observe the psychological aspects of the client (Figure 9.11).

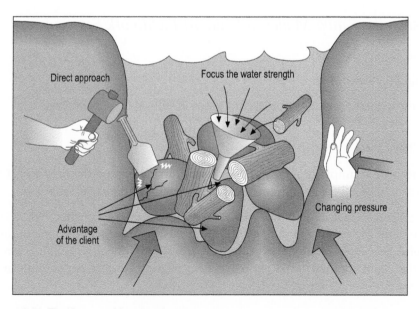

Figure 9.11 The Kawa model approach.

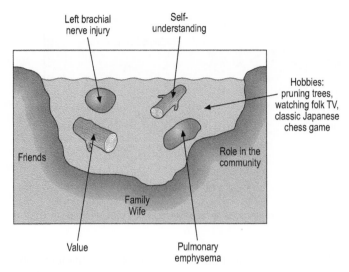

Figure 9.12 The Kawa model highlights those factors that reflect a deeper, wider understanding of the client.

To compare (1) to (2), those factors that reflect a deeper, wider, understanding of the client are highlighted:

- In (1) the main focus is on the physical functions and to find strategies

- In (2) it is possible to express the role of OT to support the client experiencing disabilities.

The Kawa model highlights those factors that reflect a deeper, wider understanding of the client (Figure 9.12):

- Psychological aspects or inner problems that are influenced by and also influence the environment or circumstances can be better appreciated through the Kawa diagrams

- The concept of self-awareness and values of the client are appreciated

- The relation between the family, health care staff and the client can also be understood and appreciated (Fig. 9.13)

- The students' values and views of life are shown in the model. This helps the supervisor to use appropriate guidance for the student

- The student becomes aware of him/herself in the client's environment and, through the process, is reminded to reflect on his or her own situation in and with the environment.

All the students who had finished their fieldwork were instructed to use the Kawa model. The students' lasting impressions of the Kawa model were:

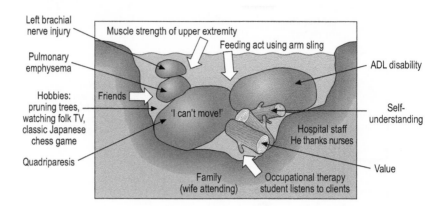

Figure 9.13 The Kawa model functions to help reveal a holistic view of client in context.

- The model helps to integrate information such as: impairments, environment, personality, psychological state, occupational therapy approaches and assets, to understand the relations and to see the client as a whole

- The model can look at the clients' situations chronologically in context, informing the occupational therapy student of the importance of clients' personal traits and social backgrounds

- The familiarity of the river as a metaphor for one's life makes imagining one's life circumstances, specifically and appropriately, much easier

- People have different values, disabilities and environments shaped by uniquely configured contexts and this can be shown in the different sizes of the structures that determine the flow of water. Again, the familiar metaphor is mutually easy for client and student to understand and share

- Students found the driftwood and spaces in the Kawa metaphor particularly difficult to comprehend and put to use. This may be due to a lack of adult life experience to reflect on in understanding the potential and effect of transient life factors.

Final Thoughts Regarding the Kawa Model as a Teaching Tool

In fieldwork education in Japan today, many students are not able to answer which models they use in their practice. They do, however, learn a significant amount of what occupational therapy practice is from their clinical experiences. The supervisors do not use specific models either, but they guide the students with what they have learned from experience. Therefore, it is necessary to make their occupational therapy practice models clearer and relevant to their own views of the world in which they live and practise.

Explaining Occupational Therapy to Health Teams; Benefits of a Culturally Relevant Occupational Therapy Model

Mie Nishihama OTR,

Staff Occupational Therapist

Shigei Hospital, Kurashiki, Japan

Hiroko Fujimoto MscOT, OTR (then of Asahigawa Jidouin Hospital for Children) aided in the translation and preparation of the author's Japanese manuscript into English. Currently, Ms Fujimoto is affiliated with the Makibi Hospital in Okayama, Japan, and Aino University Osaka, Japan

Overview

In many Japanese medical-oriented treatment facilities, the reductionistic medical model predominates in categorising client problems according to specific parts. In Japan, it is not unusual for ward staff, such as nurses or care workers, to interpret occupational therapy as 'functional training' and 'physical therapy'. Further, cooperation between health team members is often fragmented and organised with each group focusing on different parts of the client. Occupational therapy models which focus on *occupation* in contexts of the 'whole person' are largely inadequate in Japan because they reflect Western cultural patterns and meanings of what constitutes a whole person. Japanese patterns appear to favour broader, collective constructions of self and others, including the client's family and social contacts, set in the flow of time – like a river. Japanese occupational therapists have been at a loss in trying to delineate their role and practice partly due to the lack of culturally appropriate theoretical frameworks.

Most of the applications of the Kawa model thus far have been on individual clients. A clinical case from the Japanese context is used to examine whether the recently introduced 'River model' of Japanese occupational therapy is effective in explaining occupational therapy to team members and clients (Figure 9.14).

Purpose

The purpose of this inquiry was to determine whether members of the other health teams could understand the occupational therapy role in a rehabilitation setting through the Kawa model.

Method

The lead investigator initially gave an in-service presentation on the topic of 'activities of daily living (ADL) in the hospital ward'. The Kawa model was part of the presentation. Three participants in the in-service, among 12 non-OT staff

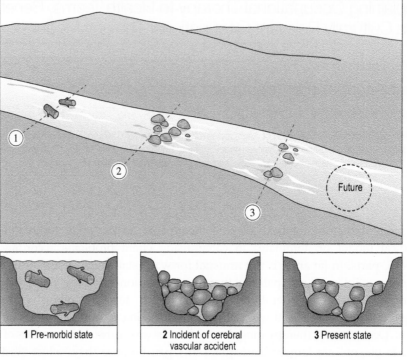

1 Pre-morbid state   **2** Incident of cerebral vascular accident   **3** Present state

Figure 9.14 Nishihama's simple diagram of a river, to explain occupational therapy to fellow health team members.

who showed interest in the topic, were chosen for a series of focused interviews.

The information below briefly describes this sample, and is arranged according to their initials, age, sex, profession, and years of work experience:

- HM: 23; female; licensed carer (kaigo-fukushi-shi); 3 years
- AT: 28; female; care assistant (kaigo-joshu); 1 year
- YW: 23; female; registered nurse; 3 years.

The following procedure was adopted for deriving information about the qualities of the Kawa model in explaining occupational therapy and its role in rehabilitation:

1 The participants were asked the question: 'What is occupational therapy?'

2 The researcher explains the Kawa model by using a case example. This explanation was limited to a mere 5 minutes, maximum

3 The participants were interviewed about their impressions on the model

4 The interviews were transcribed and analysed.

Brief Summaries of Outcomes

HM – Licensed Carer

Before the interview, HM held the impression that occupational therapists helped people to make their activities of daily living (ADLs) go more smoothly. She remarked positively often about the visual impact of the model. Talking about the model resulted in HM wanting to talk about particular problems that occupational therapy ought to address, even though she was not an occupational therapist, herself.

It became apparent that the Kawa model was not just promising for understanding the client, but it appeared to be a good tool to think about the situation and circumstances of the health professional, as well. In other words, the metaphor of the river for occupation and life flow was simple and powerful enough, even for non-occupational therapists. Non-occupational therapists, including clients, are readily enabled to imagine their own situations from an occupational perspective.

It was interesting to draw the metaphorical Kawa model in a collective process. In this way, the diverse team could examine shared meanings, similarities and differences in their professional mandates.

After the process, HM reported that her view of the occupational therapy's philosophy, view of the client and scope of practice expanded beyond ADLs.

AT – Care Assistant

Before the interview, AT held that occupational therapists helped people improve their ADL performance, physical and psychological well-being, and assist the client to return to their pre-morbid lifestyle and abilities.

When placing herself in the context of the social environment (the river floor), she placed her social status hierarchically below the occupational therapist.

Before discussing the Kawa model, AT mainly talked about the present. After the explanation, however, her perspective expanded to the client's future and goals.

Unlike the occupational therapists' focus on enhancing flow of the water by enabling the client's adaptation of the rocks and floor of the river, AT did not know what the carers' roles were in the model.

As the interview proceeded, the interviewee started to use the words and concepts from the Kawa model when discussing the client's case.

After learning the Kawa model, AT reported that her image of occupational therapy extended further into matters of the client's social and physical environment and future.

流

YW – Registered Nurse

YW's image before the interview was that occupational therapists assisted people achieve daily living function.

YW remarked that compared to the nurses' records written in words, the model can show problems in ADL and its relationships to contextual factors. It can be understood visually. She was surprised to know that occupational therapists evaluated the client's situation and context in detail in order to make their assessments of the client.

YW remarked that nurses are very busy and usually see only the surface of the client's life. 'We have not enough information about all the structures of the patient's *river.*'

She also commented that the ageing population does not have identity – that not many people pay attention to their individual needs and identity. YW agreed that their lives can each be shown and appreciated through the Kawa metaphor.

After the process, YW reported that her image of occupational therapy had expanded to include a positive regard for the client's character and adaptive assets.

Discussion

Before the Kawa model emerged, occupational therapists were largely seen as people who helped ameliorate functional disabilities, problems encountered during hospital admission, and difficulties with ADLs. After learning about occupational therapy using the Kawa model, their viewpoint and regard for occupational therapy expanded to include the client's social and physical environment, assets, and future needs of the client.

The Kawa model is stripped of theoretical jargon, presented as a simple drawing, making it easier for people to understand more about occupational therapy. The model proved to be a good vehicle to expand the usual problem-oriented discourse of the hospital setting to issues of client assets and abilities, taking into account the client's broader social and physical context of daily life. The Kawa model in this application also looked promising in regard to explicating occupational therapists' perspectives, roles and clinical realities. There was unanimous support and encouragement to use this model for the purpose of understanding and assisting the client better.

Outcomes

1 The three participants understood and related well with the Kawa model in this brief study

2 The Kawa model could be used as a means to draw out the opinions and the values of the interviewee, thus it may be a good way to facilitate ideas exchange and information among the members of the health team

3 Many of the participants in the broad in-service expressed interest in the Kawa model and gained new insight into the potential for the occupational therapy role.

The Kawa model can easily be understood with a short explanation. It can be used as a tool to understand each other's values and perspectives on life issues. In further use of the model, we would like to explore whether the concepts used in the Kawa model can be effectively used when discussing client issues in staff conferences across disciplines.

Using the Kawa Model with Occupational Therapy Students to Help Gain Insights into Working with Indigenous Australians

Alison Nelson Bocc Thy, Mocc Thy

Occupational Therapy Consultant

The Aboriginal and Torres Strait Islander Independent Community School, Brisbane, Australia

Clinical Educator and Lecturer

University of Queensland, Brisbane, Australia

Description of the Use of Kawa Model

The model was used to help first year occupational therapy students, situated in an urban Australian setting, explore issues of culture and context when working with Indigenous Australians. This was done in the context of a tutorial to support a lecture on culture and occupation. Approximately 30 students were divided into groups of three and each group was given a different case to work on. Two case examples (1 adult and 1 child) were about Indigenous Australians with whom occupational therapists may work (Figure 9.15). A third case scenario was about a non-Indigenous occupational therapy student who encountered the Indigeous client while on practicum (Figure 9.16).

Students were introduced to the Kawa model and then asked to 'make' the model for each of their cases out of materials provided to them. The materials used were play-dough (which is a kind of Plasticine material frequently used by children during play), collage materials or blocks. Students were encouraged to identify what each of their items in their river represented and then

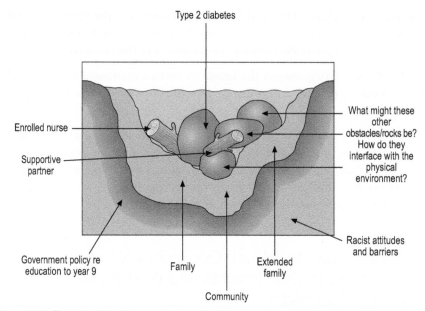

Figure 9.15 Example of the Kawa model used for the purpose of examining one of three cases relating to the occupational therapy care of Indigenous Australians.

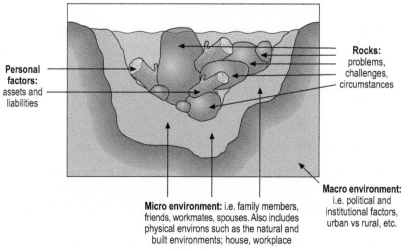

Figure 9.16 Employing the Kawa model framework to enable occupational therapy students to explore their own cultural contexts and construction of self.

give feedback to the whole class about their model. The students who constructed 'their river' had to also identify what 'bridges' they could form between their own river and their client's river in order to provide appropriate and meaningful occupational therapy services.

Outcomes and Insights

Students embraced the use of a 'hands-on' activity and developed some spectacular models. They were able to use the model to identify potential assets, liabilities and problems in each scenario. They generally had much greater difficulty identifying these issues for their own river than for their clients. Some of these student groups used the collage materials to adapt the model from a river to 'their story' with pictures and other objects depicting different parts of their lives. The model enabled them to see the client in his/her entire context rather than separating out issues of 'culture' from those related to the presenting clinical concern.

Some students appeared to have difficulty separating the environmental context from the assets or liabilities when they were related to the client's social context, for example, a caring partner could form both part of the environmental context and an asset.

When asked about how to build bridges between the two rivers, students identified that the primary way of doing this was through developing an effective relationship. They also identified that they would need to be confident in their clinical skills and knowledge in being able to place these in the client's context and understanding. While this was done at a fairly basic level, it was a useful exploration for students in only their first year of occupational therapy studies.

Students' feedback about the exercise was overwhelmingly positive with many students noting that the model helped to identify client's goals and gain their perspective; that it was dynamic; that it enabled the therapist to see the interrelationship between all the parts of a person's life; that it was holistic; that it was easy to visualise and they could see themselves using it with a client. One student reported that he found it difficult to make the links between the different parts of the model.

One particular comment about the use of the model showed a depth of insight:

> It helped me see that not everything has to be perfect in a client's life (i.e. that the person did not have to be 'fixed' but rather empowered to overcome obstacles and that if some of the issues were out of the way then that could increase a person's quality of life).

Overall I found this exercise to be extremely valuable in helping the students gain a broader understanding of Indigenous Australians in their contexts and to begin to explore how their own 'river' has an impact on their interactions with and occupational therapy service provision for Indigenous Australians.

REFERENCES

[1] Hagedorn R. Foundations for Practice in Occupational Therapy. Edinburgh: Churchill Livingstone; 2001

[2] Lim KH, Iwama M. Emerging models – an Asian perspective: the Kawa model. In: Duncan E (ed.), Foundations for Practice in Occupational Therapy. Edinburgh: Churchill Livingstone; 2005

[3] World Health Organization. International Classification of Impairments, Disabilities, and Handicaps. Geneva: ICF; 1980

[4] World Health Organization. International Classification of Functioning, Disability and Health. Geneva: ICF; 2001

Towards Culturally Relevant and Safe Theory in Occupational Therapy

The Kawa model constitutes a novel addition to the progression of occupational therapy theory development in a number of ways. Students of theory in occupational therapy, in reading through these chapters, may have marked and reflected on some of the features and characteristics that separate the Kawa model from other, more established, conceptual models. Some of these points of distinction and comparison are raised here for the purpose of further reflection and to enlighten occupational therapists towards new ways of considering theory from a cultural perspective. Cultural comparisons not only enable a more profound understanding of a model's structure and language. Comparative analyses can also function to illuminate the features of familiar models and theory, and raise what had previously remain hidden or taken for granted, to new possibilities of insight and application.

Some Distinctive Features of the Kawa Model

One of the most distinct and important features of the Kawa model is its regard as a culturally relevant and *safe* work, having been raised originally from the Japanese social context, using concepts drawn from the Japanese lexicon aligned in a structure that diverges from familiar scientific and rational form. 'Kawa' is the Japanese word for 'river', and is a familiar metaphor for 'life'. Readers may have wondered whether this metaphor could qualify as a theoretical model, given its unfamiliar structure and departure from conventional linear-logical form. When considered against the features and functions becoming of theoretical frameworks mentioned in Chapter 2 – that theory serves to describe, explain, validate[1], guide[2] and predict[3] processes of occupational therapy – then the Kawa model qualifies as a theoretical work.

Readers may readily associate some of the model's features, particularly its reliance on a metaphor of nature, to Eastern philosophical elements observable in Buddhist (particularly related to but not limited to Mahayana and Zen) ideologies as well as from Confucian and Taoist ethics, but ultimately the associations will vary inevitably according to the cultural lenses of its appraisers[4]. Although the original concepts are labelled with Japanese terms, the concepts can be renamed to suit the client's lexicon and associated meanings. This is an important point of distinction that carries significant implications for client-centred application. With respect to applying the Kawa model, the client's experiences are not required to be translated nor transformed to suit someone else's lexicon and rigidly defined concepts. The rocks, river sides and walls, driftwood and water become the categories through which the client expresses his or her issues of daily living in proper and relevant context. There is a significant shift in power relation as it is the client who names and constructs the meanings of each concept. The principles that form between the concepts are then also named and explained by the client. As stated earlier, as with the use of all conceptual models, when and if the metaphor and its framework of possible meanings does not fit the client's contexts of realities, the model should be put aside for alternatives that do not disadvantage the client nor skew the client's narratives of occupation.

Readers would have also noticed that the Kawa model was raised from the clinical practice context through naturalistic/qualitative means, involving practitioners (and their clients) who had limited postgraduate academic experience. This is not the usual origin or the way in which conventional conceptual models have been developed in our profession. The clinical context may have been the source of inspiration, the place where the theorists amassed their practice experiences, as well as the appropriate place where theory is to be refined, but rarely before has a model been *actually* raised from practice. The bottom-up dynamic for theory development is not so novel in other disciplines, but the manner and dynamic by which the Kawa model was raised is new to occupational therapy. Thus the model is grounded in and inspired by the realities of occupational therapy practice. It should be primarily evaluated according to its utility and meaning in the practice context.

Another distinctive feature of the Kawa model can be found in its structure. The inner framework and dynamics of the model diverge from conventional quantitative theory in its departure from a linear, directional form. Explanatory frameworks that are based on mathematical and physical logic are often challenged when employed with purpose to explain universally the complexities of subjective human experience and matters of phenomenological meaning. Matters of 'being', 'occupation', or the concept of spirituality, as examples, with their complex cultural constructions extend beyond the predictive limits of empirical theory. Since the dawn of the industrial age, the machine has emerged as a popular metaphor to describe and explain humans and human experience. In our ascent into the age of information, simple machines have yielded to complex mechanicals and 'systems'. The Kawa model does not participate in any unconscious attempt to take all that is natural, complex and unfathomably particular as the human experience and reduce it to finite, relatively narrow mechanical depictions. The Kawa model is devoid of explicit, rigid, universal postulates. There are no discrete boxes connected by linear, directional arrows, nor is there any reliance on rational, artificial, mechanical metaphors (such as 'systems') to explain its dynamic. The complex, profound, interweaving of self and nature, that forms the bases on which meanings are ascribed to occupations in Eastern world views require a flexible, particular and responsive dynamic. The Kawa model's departure from conventional scientific form will likely draw criticism from empirically oriented observers but its unconventional structure may paradoxically represent the model's strength.

Ascribing to a more natural, cosmological and ontological basis to viewing 'self' as embedded in the environment rather than in a more rational construction of self opposed, vis-à-vis the environment, the model does not subsume nor feature a discrete, centrally situated self. Self is decentralised and embedded in contexts of time, space and within all other components of an inseparable environment. Harmony and balance in this fluid, comprehensive sense is not based on individual determinism or causation but on all elements that form the context of human experience. This does not disqualify the Kawa model for clients situated in a culture that leans towards individualism. On the contrary, the Kawa model encourages a client-centred perspective by bringing in and giving greater weight to the unique contextual circumstances in which the client is situated. The self as embedded in nature provides another vantage from which to look at clients in a broader context. The Kawa model has enabled some occupational therapists in the West to appreciate that an (over)emphasis on a centrally situated individual can effect a subtle de-emphasis of the environment in relation to the self. The complexity of components that make up the rich context in which meanings in occupations are dependent, become as important as self in the framework of the Kawa model.

Another feature of the model and one that needs to be explored further is its relational qualities that appear to render the model as useful when applied to individuals as well as to collectives. The emphasis on occupations from an individual experience vantage has consequently been a limiting factor when attempting to expand occupational therapy's possibilities into the realm of non-Western social contexts. Some models can be 'bent' to accommodate family in lieu of a single client, but rarely have we observed these narratives of occupation taken beyond the individual families to organisations like companies, or a particular social process – like 'alleviating barriers to occupational justice' in a given setting. For this example, the idea of occupational justice makes up the river, while the river walls and sides might be the social and institutional context, and rocks of various sizes comprising the barriers. Readers are encouraged to try the model on a variety of situations and examine the model's utility and potential in this respect. Instead of an individual client being the subject of the river, why not a family, or organisation (like your occupational therapy association), company, or an entire community? When occupation is conceptualised in a way that does not limit it to the individual, we are afforded a window into new possibilities and ways to evaluate the current construction of occupation, as occupational therapists have known it. Over the past 5 years, case studies of the model's application across the spectrum from neonatal to end of life, from individuals to organisations and communities, and across the medical categories of rehabilitation and mental health, have been collected[5].

Intended to be culturally relevant, all universal premises of the Kawa model and its applicability are dismissed, availing the model to alteration in conceptual and structural ways by clients and occupational therapists to match the specific social and cultural contexts of their diverse clientele. Although the model may appear to favour Japanese cultural contexts, the

Kawa model should not be viewed as culturally exclusive. The utility of this model for varying populations depends on the river metaphor's relevance to its subjects. Since the model was introduced outside of Japan[6,7,8,9,10,11,12,13,14], groups of practitioners in other cultural locations spanning four continents have begun to use the model, adapting it freely to suit the cultural requirements and unique features of their practice. The model should be employed as a tool to understand better and appreciate the complex occupational worlds from the client's viewpoints, and never as a universal framework brought to bear on compliant, subordinated clients.

A Matter of Culturally Safe Conceptual Models

In various parts of this book, issues have been raised about the 'cultural safety' of the Kawa model and other theoretical material. Nurse and health scholars from Aotearoa (Maori term for New Zealand) in the last two decades have stressed the importance of *cultural safety*[15,16]. Cultural safety is a framework by which power relationships between health professionals and the peoples they serve are critically considered. Maori health scholars have examined the impact of historical, social, and political processes on minority health disparities in Aotearoa and these imperatives have now extended to global contexts where equity is of interest wherever health issues of a particular group are being described, mediated and evaluated by other people and their foreign cultural standards. The idea of cultural safety is especially pertinent to occupational therapists at this point in time as our long held universal assumptions and practices continue to transcend cultural boundaries in places and people outside of the cultural contexts where the ideas originated. The basic example given earlier was of the social imperatives of autonomy, self-efficacy, unilateral determinism (entitled control of the environment) and equality, brought to bear on people socialised into collectivist, interdependent, and hierarchically organised shared experiences. Often the recipients have yet to develop the necessary abilities to evaluate critically imported ideologies and methods and stand to be discriminated against further by standards and norms belonging to a different context. The ability to exercise critical evaluation, in the Western sense of it, requires the acquisition of rational analytical methods that are further supported in the contexts of Western social life and education. As mentioned previously, these materials, including theory in particular, take on an aura of having descended from heaven and assume a kind of authoritative status. For these and similar reasons, the theory and epistemology of occupational therapy have rarely been brought under the disrespecting scrutiny of a critical lens. The unfamiliarity with and inability to exercise rational thinking – the very bases on which theory and conceptual models are constructed – stand in the way of any cogent attempt to determine the veracity, utility and *cultural safety* of the material.

Determining Cultural Safety: Some Points to Ponder

In order to determine the relative cultural safety of theoretical material before it is applied to a particular population, the following guiding questions are offered. This is not an exhaustive set of cues by any means, but they should give the culturally sensitive practitioner some direction and a sense of what cultural safety in theory application might entail.

Starting with language, what needs to be determined is whether the actual words and concepts contained in the model make sense to the client. Does the language disadvantage the client in any way? Power is often exercised in a subtle way. It is interesting to examine how many patients of modern medicine do not understand the medical explanations and meanings of the diagnoses applied to them. Though the condition or diagnoses may be about the patient, there is often some fear involved on the patient's part in asking the professional, who is regarded to be more knowledgeable about matters of health, to explain the situation in clear, understandable terms – to translate the terms germane to the culture of professional medicine, to the culture of the patient. The meanings of a person's occupations are unique and particular to the client's sphere of experiences: the client knows best, in the frame of occupational therapy. Are the concepts of the model written in the client's lexicon? If the words have been translated into the client's lexicon, do they remain valid in the client's social context? Are the concepts and principles that purportedly tie them together comprehensible in proper context to both client and therapist? Any shortcoming in the client's comprehension of the processes that he or she is a participant may translate into an imbalance of power, and depending on cultural norms, this may be a point of concern. The worst possible case, in a Western context, can occur when the client is being led through a therapeutic process in which he or she does not understand nor comprehend, but feels too intimidated and disempowered to halt the process. No degree of comments like: 'Don't worry, I am the professional and I know what's best for you', is acceptable or assuring in such cases.

Occupational therapy has always been about enabling our clients to participate in what is meaningful to them. If so, then the issue of culture, in the broader sense described in this book, is fundamental to the development of knowledge and theory in this profession. In terms of theory, some very difficult questions and challenging issues then arise. How do we justify taking our client's narratives and issues pertaining to what they see as meaningful engagement and force or translate these into the structure, language and professional ideology of another, seemingly universal view of normal? As we proceed to deliver occupational therapy in varying cultural contexts, we cannot assume that client-centred practice is actually happening. Merely asking the client about issues of occupational performance does not in itself qualify the process as being client centred. Being client centred transcends the overt practice of consulting clients and giving them a primary role in selecting and directing the process, also to include the very structure and language of occupational therapy theory.

Cultural safety of models and theory are not only about the language, concepts and principles that tie them together. Occupational therapists and the client need to be aware critically of the structure of the theoretical material, where significantly powerful imperatives and cultural norms lay hidden from the obvious. The same questions raised in the preceding paragraph about the language of models need to be asked of theory structure. Social structural norms, such as individualism, egalitarianism, rationalism, the location and construction of 'self', the environment and what constitutes the relationship between the two, as well as narratives of disablement and well-being, are all embedded here. Much of the content of the earlier and middle chapters of this book were purposely put together with the intent of displaying these subtle but extremely important considerations. These features are discernable by asking some simple questions of a given model. How is the self represented and how is self constructed? What does the structure tell you about the nature of the relationship between self and other entities like the environment? Where and how are these entities located? A centrally placed individual and an environment placed in the periphery but given less space or prominence vis-à-vis the self, speaks volumes about the underlying assumptions of the model. Does the model accommodate collectives, family and community as well as it does matters relating to the individual? The concern for cultural safety is summarised by the following final question: 'Are the narratives of occupation, well-being and disablement consistent with the client and therapist's comprehension of the same, and do these agree with the local cultural context?' The degree with which these structural factors agree with the client and therapist's view of the world and shared meanings, will influence to a great degree the cultural safety of the theoretical material to the world of the client.

The Kawa model represents a controversial work. Until now, most of our theory has come from contexts removed from the realities and shared experienced of the clinician and client. It has been a 'top-down' affair in a professional context in which the perceived gap between academicians and clinicians continues to widen. What the profession needs now is theory based on the specific contexts of occupational therapy practice. In the pursuit of scientific legitimacy, the clinic as a rich context for culturally relevant and innovative ideas is in danger of being been shut out of the epistemological and theoretical discourse of this profession.

Culture: The Confluence of Ideas in Occupational Therapy

Theoretical material as we have studied it in Western contexts and classrooms can carry an aura of difficulty – of being detached from reality and actual practice, of being comprised of esoteric language and of being incomprehensible to clients. This image of theory in our ranks seems to contradict theory's merits and purposes – to take complex phenomena and objects in our world of experience and reduce them to simpler, comprehensible descriptions or explanations. If the occupational therapist cannot grasp and understand a particular theoretical work or material, he or she should hold the self-berating for another time. Examine the theoretical work carefully and consider whether the problem might reside in the theory itself.

The Japanese occupational therapy clinicians who embarked on the path to raise the Kawa model from their practice contexts were buoyed by a realisation that their shortcomings in comprehending and applying conceptual models imported from the West, lay more in the models rather than to some inadequacy of intellect among themselves. For years, they had bought all of the translated books, attended expensive workshops, and earnestly studied contemporary models of occupational therapy, wondering why it all wasn't resonating on a deeper level. Culture is where these therapists eventually turned to search for the answers to their theoretical crises. Eventually, with the help of some cultural comparative reflection, they were able to agree that theory and knowledge construction, like their own existence, was situated in place and time, bound in the context of the theorist's views of reality. One theorist's views and constructions of 'normal' could turn out to be quite a different 'normal' from one's own, informed by a different constellation of shared experiences set in a particular place and time.

If the issues of situated meaning raised in this book carry any degree of credibility with the reader, there should be subsequent understanding that these barriers and challenges to congruence between theory and self or communities do indeed exist and the problems of comprehension are not necessarily located on one side of the theory–occupational therapist–client triangle. The problems of comprehension are located on all sides of the delta and their confluence is *culture*.

Implications for Cultural Competency

Culture represents much more than material features that distinguish people from others. The views of culture expounded on in this book through a discourse on theory and conceptual models concur that culture is just as much a dynamic process, a complex interplay of meanings that represent and shape the individual and collective lives of people, as it is about narratives of shared experiences. Until now, occupational therapists have not really taken their analyses of culture beyond 'cultural competency'[15], to consider how it is an integral part of occupational therapy's conceptual models, theory and epistemology. Therefore, when we ponder developing culturally relevant and safe models of occupational therapy, we can expect some fundamental continuity between the culture (shared meanings), ontology (views of truth) and epistemology (philosophy of knowledge) of the model constructors and their models. According to this way of knowing, occupational therapy qualifies as a cultural entity given its shared language, meanings, code of acceptable conduct, institutional standards of knowledge production and narratives (like conceptual models), etc.

Given this broadening of culture, the ubiquitous terms – cultural awareness, cultural sensitivity and cultural competency – should perhaps be re-examined and conceptualised to take on broader, more equitable meanings. These terms must now include the treatment of and awareness of occupational therapy as a cultural entity and force, and expand the cultural constitution of people to transcend individual embodiment to broader dimensions of the social. Culturally aware and sensitive occupational therapists will acknowledge and honour the validity of people's diverse world views, value patterns and ways of knowing, and respect the client's right to a particular view of reality. These occupational therapists will understand their own personal cultural being, appreciate the cultural construction of occupational therapy and know that their professional practice in its conventional form, driven by a certain ideological bent may not always resonate on a more profound or fundamental level with their diverse clientele, where it really matters. Challenged and hopefully discredited to a certain degree in these chapters is the universalistic sentiment that: 'My views and values of occupation are right and therefore appropriate for all others'.

Cultural competency is cultural awareness and cultural sensitivity embodied and enacted. It begins with profound tolerance and unconditional positive regard for all clients, no matter what markers of diversity they represent or embody. The culturally competent occupational therapist is a 21st century super-hero who understands and checks his or her own person's and profession's cultural constitutions, and goes to the ends of the earth to appreciate each client without judgement and understand as much as possible the broader social context in which the client finds themselves in a position of seeking help. Cultural competence comes full circle when the occupational therapist is able to enable the client to reach a higher plane that is meaningful to the client's particular world view and sphere of meanings. In one context, that higher plane might be about enabling a greater sense of unilateral control over the environment and circumstances. In another instance, the higher plane may be about instilling a sense of harmony or balance between the client's self and circumstance. Metaphorically, this may be about walls of water bashing through dams of intertwined rocks and driftwood, or about water slipping through cracks and around the debris, in life's river. For occupational therapists to attain a more culturally competent practice, more culturally relevant theory, related tools and knowledge are required. The Kawa model is one example of the kind of theoretical model and tool that occupational therapists can choose in the quest to illuminate and understand the client better – on the client's terms.

The Kawa model was developed in response to the need for culturally relevant and safe theory, championed by clinicians who were experiencing the inequities brought about by theoretical material being systematically implemented out of cultural context. In a sense, these Asian occupational therapists were simply looking for a way to advance their occupational therapy to a higher degree of meaning and relevance. At the core of their theoretical wanderings was a mandate to better centre, adjust and fashion the form, function and meaning of occupational therapy to their client's real world of meanings. They were able to achieve this by appreciating and discerning theory and conceptual models for what they are – narratives and cultural artefacts that are situated and bound by specific cultural norms and spheres of shared experiences. They realised that the existing dominant conceptual models they learned were not necessarily bad or 'wrong'. Rather, they were able to draw a distinction from a vantage of cultural relativism that allowed them to appreciate the connection between the culturally bound meanings embedded in these imported theory and the cultural contexts in which these materials were originally raised.

How will conceptual model development and application evolve over time? As the post-modern discourses of social constructionism and cultural relativism take greater hold in the social sciences and find their way into occupational therapy, and as our core ideas become increasingly subject to more intense scrutiny from a rapidly changing global community, it might simply be a matter of time before the profession realises and embraces a more diverse and socially just regard for its theory. Theory and practice are inextricably intertwined for the successful delivery of occupational therapy. The thesis of this book has been to illuminate culture's fundamental place in the theory and practice of this wonderful profession. Occupational therapy, encompassing its constellation of theory, epistemology and practice, can be likened to a river set in the context of society. For the profession to survive and flourish, it must do so in concert with society, in a similar way to which the form, function and meanings of its structures mirrors the same of the society through which it flows, finds its shape and its bearing. In the new millennium, culture, as discoursed in these pages, presents one of occupational therapy's biggest, most important challenges and possibly its biggest asset. How the profession deals with the fundamental issue of relevance and meaning of occupation for all of its diverse clientele across cultural boundaries will determine whether occupational therapy will deliver on its magnificent promise.

And perhaps one day, and not so far in the future of this profession, occupational therapists will apply the language of the metaphors they share with their clients. Perhaps in some instances then, occupational therapy processes may commence and conclude with the simple question: 'How does your river flow?'

REFERENCES

1 Clark PN. Theoretical frameworks in contemporary occupational therapy practice, Part 1. American Journal of Occupational Therapy 1979; 33:505–514

2 Miller R. What is theory and why does it matter? In: Miller R, Sieg K, Ludwig F, Shortridge S, Van Deusen J (eds), Six Perspectives on Theory for the Practice of Occupational Therapy. Rockville: Aspen Publishers Inc; 1988

3 Duldt B, Giffin K. Theoretical Perspectives for Nursing. Boston: Little. Brown & Co; 1985

4 Lim KH, Iwama MK. Emerging models – an Asian Perspective; the Kawa (river) model. In: Duncan E (ed.), Foundations for Practice in Occupational Therapy. Edinburgh: Churchill Livingstone; 2005; 161–189

5 Hatsutori T, Hibino K, Iwama M, et al. Applications of the Kawa (river) model: findings from case studies and discussions. Singapore: 3rd Asia Pacific Occupational Therapy Congress; 2003

6 Okuda M, Iwama M, Hatsutori T, et al. A Japanese model of occupational therapy; One; the 'river model' raised from the clinical setting. Journal of the Japanese Association of Occupational Therapists 2000; 19 Supplement:512

7 Iwama M, Hatsutori T, Okuda M. Emerging a culturally and clinically relevant conceptual model of Japanese occupational therapy. Stockholm: 13th International Congress of the World Federation of Occupational Therapists; 2002

8 Hibino K, Tanaka M, Iwama M, et al. Applying a new model of Japanese occupational therapy to a client case of depression. Stockholm: 13th International Congress of the World Federation of Occupational Therapists; 2002

9 Yoshimura N, Hibino K, Iwama M. The Japanese 'Kawa' model of occupational therapy in the context of mental health. Stockholm: 13th International Congress of the World Federation of Occupational Therapists; 2002

10 Fujimoto H, Yoshimura N, Iwama M. The Kawa (river) model workshop – addressing diversity of culture in occupational therapy. Singapore: 3rd Asia Pacific Occupational Therapy Congress; 2003

11 Okuda M, Kataoka N, Takahashi H, et al. The Kawa (river) model: reflections on our culture. Singapore: 3rd Asia Pacific Occupational Therapy Congress; 2003

12 Iwama M, Fujimoto H, Townsend E. The Kawa (river) model; occupation, nature and culture flowing. Athens: 7th European Congress of Occupational Therapy. Oral Presentation, 23 September; 2004

13 Iwama M. The Kawa (river) model: the power of culturally relevant occupational therapy theory. Ergoterapeuten, the magazine of the Norwegian Occupational Therapy Association; 2005; Feb, 8–16

[14] Iwama M. The Kawa model, reconceptualizing occupational therapy. Oral presentation: invited keynote presentation, Challenge and Change. Sheffield Hallam University, Sheffield: Reconceptualising Occupational Therapy Conference; 2005; March 20

[15] Ramsden I. Kawa whakaruruhau – cultural safety in nursing education in Aotearoa: report to the Ministry of Education. Wellington: Ministry of Education; 1990

[16] Jungerson K. Culture, theory and the practice of occupational therapy in New Zealand/Aotearoa. American Journal of Occupational Therapy 1992; 46:745–750

Index

F

Face 96
Factions (*habatsu*) 67, 91
Failure 89, 142
Family ('ie') structure 84
Fate (*unme*) 26, 51
Flexible truths 85, 124, 127
Flow, water of life *see under* Life
Focal points 169
Frame *see Ba* (Frame)
Front, in (*omote*) 95, 98–99
Fudosei (climaticity) 65
Fujimoto, H. 184, 192, 205, 211
Fukei kousei hou (projection method) 141
Functional states of the individual 47, 211

G

Gender 28
General Systems Theory (GST) 47
Genghis Khan 69, 72
Give and take 64
Glaser, B. 121, 160
God 37, 63–64, 65, 112–113, 116
Greenhouse effect 43
Grounded Theory 121, 123, 128
    methodology 126
    modified 131
    process 141
Group 51, 61, 82, 83
    aspirations 96
    harmony 81
    identity 86
    orientation 81
    self-in-relation-to- 84
    social 64
    structure 69
Guatemalan immigrants 181
Guilt 64
Gustafson, J.M. 65

H

Habatsu (factions) 67, 91
Habituation 47
Haga, Y. 62
Hagedorn, R. 179
Hamaguchi, E. 63
Handicap *see* Disability
Hands energized by mind and will 12, 104
Hara (abdomen) 98
Harmony 72, 188
    balance, control and 161–164
    collective 69, 81, 117, 192–197
    nature and 102, 116, 142–143
    personal attributes and 73–75
Hatsutori, T. 130, 205

Health 120, 130, 206
    illness and 95, 124
    teams 211–215
Heaven's punishment (*bachi*) 63
Hendry, J. 67, 82, 94
'Here and now' existence 62, 66, 175
Hierarchy 101
    in Japanese history 82–83
    political 95
    relationships and 90–94
        inverted 'V' 90–91
    social view in 118
    structures of 103, 105
Hindu caste system 81
Hito (others) 97–98
'Ho-Jo-Ki' (Kamono) 140
Hobbes, T. 102
Holistic approach 147, 153, 172–173, 184, 211
Hong Kong 22
Honne (inner truth) 67, 95, 98–99
Horizontal
    indexing 95–97, 115
    social structure 97–99
Household ('ie') structure 84
Human relations (*ningen-kankai*) 85–87, 103, 105, 131
    in vertically structured society 67
Humans, cosmology and nature 65–66

I

Ideas 37, 226–227
Identity 88–89
    crises 117–121, 124
    doing and 62, 115
    group 86
    personal 86, 186
'Ie' (family) structure 84–85
Ijime (bullying) 89
illness *see* disability; health
Impairment *see* Disability
Impotence 148
Independence 41, 82, 192–197
Indexing 101, 115
India 94–95
Individualism 36–38, 44–45, 64, 81, 132, 187
    Western 36–38, 112–114
Individuals 48
    analytic 44, 113
    determinism 145
    egocentric 81
    functional states 47, 211
    orientation 81
    race and ethnicity 6–7
Industrialised societies 43
Inen (karma) 63
Informed consent 82
Inner truth (*honne*) 67, 95, 98–99

Index